SpringerBriefs in Population Studies

Population Studies of Japan

The world population is expected to expand by 39.4 % to 9.6 billion in 2060 (UN World Population Prospects, revised 2010). Meanwhile, Japan is expected to see its population contract by nearly one-third to 86.7 million, and its proportion of the elderly (65 years of age and over) will account for no less than 39.9 % (National Institute of Population and Social Security Research in Japan, Population Projections for Japan 2012). Japan has entered the post-demographic transitional phase and will be the fastest shrinking country in the world, followed by former Eastern bloc nations, leading other Asian countries that are experiencing drastic changes.

A declining population that is rapidly aging impacts a country's economic growth, labor market, pensions, taxation, health care, and housing. The social structure and geographical distribution in the country will drastically change, and short-term as well as long-term solutions for economic and social consequences of this trend will be required.

This series aims to draw attention to Japan's entering the post-demographic transition phase and to present cutting-edge research in Japanese population studies. It will include compact monographs under the editorial supervision of the Population Association of Japan (PAJ).

The PAJ was established in 1948 and organizes researchers with a wide range of interests in population studies of Japan. The major fields are (1) population structure and aging; (2) migration, urbanization, and distribution; (3) fertility; (4) mortality and morbidity; (5) nuptiality, family, and households; (6) labor force and unemployment; (7) population projection and population policy (including family planning); and (8) historical demography. Since 1978, the PAJ has been publishing the academic journal *Jinkogaku Kenkyu* (The Journal of Population Studies), in which most of the articles are written in Japanese.

Thus, the scope of this series spans the entire field of population issues in Japan, impacts on socioeconomic change, and implications for policy measures. It includes population aging, fertility and family formation, household structures, population health, mortality, human geography and regional population, and comparative studies with other countries.

This series will be of great interest to a wide range of researchers in other countries confronting a post-demographic transition stage, demographers, population geographers, sociologists, economists, political scientists, health researchers, and practitioners across a broad spectrum of social sciences.

More information about this series at http://www.springer.com/series/13101

Yukiko Senda

Childbearing and Careers of Japanese Women Born in the 1960s

A Life Course That Brought Unintended Low Fertility

Springer

Yukiko Senda
Department of Liberal Arts
Tohoku Gakuin University
Sendai, Miyagi
Japan

ISSN 2211-3215 ISSN 2211-3223 (electronic)
SpringerBriefs in Population Studies
ISSN 2198-2724 ISSN 2198-2732 (electronic)
Population Studies of Japan
ISBN 978-4-431-55065-5 ISBN 978-4-431-55066-2 (eBook)
DOI 10.1007/978-4-431-55066-2

Library of Congress Control Number: 2015938732

Springer Tokyo Heidelberg New York Dordrecht London

Printed on acid-free paper

Springer Japan KK is part of Springer Science+Business Media
(www.springer.com)

Preface

This book provides the keys to understanding the trajectory that Japanese society has followed toward its very low fertility since the 1980s. The focus is on characteristics of the life course of women born in the 1960s. They are the first cohort to show the decline in marriage which causes low fertility. This book explores the experiences of the 1960s cohort of Japanese women and the factors determining their choices in their life course.

After the 1980s, drastic changes in the demographic and socioeconomic circumstances altered the Japanese family formation patterns, working conditions of young people, and public opinions and social norms on work, family, and life course. This trend started when the 1960s cohort graduated school, appeared in the labor market, and entered in the stage of family formation. Labor law amendments illegalized gender discrimination, calling public attention to gender equality and the work-family interface issued in workplaces. Japanese workplaces developed a so-called course-based human resource management system, which was substantially gender based, and brought about some changes in women's career development by treating most of them as so-called *ippan-shoku* (general clerical workers not eligible for executive positions).

These changes in circumstances for women's work, along with the loosening of social norms on the timing of major life events, created a new possibility in women's life course choice. Continue working instead of getting married and leaving the labor market in their early 20s became a real option for them. Some of them stayed single, or married in the later stages of their life, or postponed the timing to have children. Childbearing thus shifted to later stages of their life course. As a result, the current average age of pregnancy is approaching the biological limit and unintended infertility is increasing due to postponed pregnancy.

This book explores the links between the changes in social/demographic conditions and individuals' experiences of the 1960s cohort. Chapters 2 and 3 outlined the changes in Japanese society from the perspectives of demographic conditions (Chap. 2) and from law, norm, and social institutions (Chap. 3), based on quantitative data. Chapters 4 and 5 describe individuals' experiences in workplaces under course-based management systems since the 1980s (Chap. 4) and struggles to reconcile work with family responsibility (Chap. 5), mainly based on qualitative interview data.

The 1960s cohort represents a new life course pattern of Japanese women. It has been shaped through individual choices under the social structure, which still exists in Japanese society today. The experiences of the 1960s cohort women are thus the key to understanding current social/demographic problems in Japan.

Yukiko Senda

Acknowledgments

I would like to express my sincere thanks to all the individuals and organizations that have supported me.

First of all, I would like to give my deep gratitude to the surveyed subjects who voluntarily joined this study. Without their commitment, nothing could have been started. They participated in the study because they wanted to change Japanese society in light of their experiences in such a way as to allow individuals to live their lives in a better way. I hope this book has some effect in achieving that goal.

I am also very grateful to Dr. Shigesato Takahashi, because he gave me the chance to join in the Research on Policy Planning and Evaluation/Health Labour Sciences Research Grant (H20-Seisaku-Ippan-008). In this research project, Dr. Takahashi, along with the other research members, gave me valuable advice. I learned very much from this research and truly appreciate their advice.

I express my thanks to Dr. Miho Iwasawa, who kindly and carefully indicated the points of my study that should be improved. Her comments helped me a great deal.

I am also very grateful to Dr. Akiko Ouchi, because she invited me to participate in a collaborative study on female workers under the course-based management system. She studied the so-called *sogo-shoku* employees, while I studied the so-called *ippan-shoku* employees. The revised results of my part of the collaborative study are shown in Study 2, Chap. 4.

In addition, I am thankful to Dr. Sigeto Tanaka. He spared no effort in helping me with my study.

Finally, I would like to express my deepest gratitude to the late Dr. Shojiro Takao. He led me by the hand to advance on the first step to becoming a researcher.

Some parts of this book were made possible by grants issued for studies. Chapter 2 is based on a study conducted as part of the Research on Policy Planning and Evaluation/Health Labour Sciences Research Grant (H20-Seisaku-Ippan-008).

Study 1 in Chap. 4 is based on a study funded by a grant from the Tokyo Josei Zaidan. Study 3 in Chap. 4 is based on a study funded by a grant from JSPS Kakenhi 13730093. Chapter 5 is based on a study conducted as part of the Research on Policy Planning and Evaluation/Health Labour Sciences Research Grant (H14-Seisaku-029).

Yukiko Senda

Contents

Chapter 1
Introduction

This book intends to portray the characteristics of the life course of Japanese women by focusing on the 1960s cohort (the birth cohort of the 1960s). I focus on this cohort because the cohort total fertility rate (CTFR) for this cohort sharply declined (Suzuki 2013). I will look at the social conditions that led to this decline, examining them from the standpoint of women's experience. The theoretical perspectives introduced in this discussion are the life course perspective, career development perspective, and work-family interface perspective.

First, I will briefly describe the modern history of Japan that leads to today's low fertility. Since the late 20th century, the fertility rate has been consistently falling in Japanese society. However, the nature of this demographic shift differs considerably between the period lasting from the 1950s through the 1970s, and the time after 1980. From the 1950s through the 1970s, the decline was mainly due to the decrease in the marital fertility rate, which itself resulted from the spread of contraception and induced abortion (Aoki 1970). This can be regarded as part of the common process of demographic transition (Institute for International Cooperation, Japan International Corporation Agency 2003) that occurred upon modernisation. In contrast, fertility declined since the 1980s because of the decline in marriage and the increased rate of late marriage (Hirosima 2001; Iwasawa 2008). In other words, it was due to an increased deviation from the 'standard' life course of marrying and having children while young (Ochiai 1997). Changes in the structure of reproduction due to deviations from the standard life course have been observed in many developed societies. Such phenomenon is often referred to as 'the second demographic transition' (Van de Kaa 1987).

Immediately after Japan's defeat in World War II, there was a marriage rush due to marriages that were deferred during the war and the subsequent first baby boom (1947–1949) in Japan. The net reproduction rate (NRR) during this period ranged between 1.68 and 1.75 (Yamaguchi and Yajima 1973).

Shortly after that came a period of sharp decline in fertility (Honda 1962; Tachi 1969; Aoki 1970). Because of the war, the real national income per capita fell by half of the pre-war level (Cabinet Office 1955). In these extreme economic difficulties, families had to limit their number of children. During this period, the

Y. Senda, *Childbearing and Careers of Japanese Women Born in the 1960s*,
Population Studies of Japan, DOI 10.1007/978-4-431-55066-2_1

primary measure behind the reduced number of children was the popularisation of contraception. Only 28.6 % of married couples used contraception in 1950 (Mainichi Newspapers Population Problems Research Council 2000). In 1952, The Ministry of Welfare attempted to popularise birth control through contraception by issuing guidelines for popularising birth control (Koseisho Ei-hatsu No. 585, dated 27 June 1952). As a result, 62.7 % of married couples were using contraception by 1960 (Mainichi Newspapers Population Problems Research Council 2000). Another method was to induce abortion, in which the pregnancy is artificially terminated by medical measures. After the Eugenic Protection Act legalised abortion in 1947, the use of induced abortion to limit the number of children increased (Okazaki 1955). For example, in 1955, the number of induced abortions was extremely high, at 67.6 per 100 births (Aoki 1970).

By 1957, the NRR had fallen below 1, to 0.92. Population falls when the NRR is less than 1; therefore, there was already a sign of Japan's declining population during this period. Japan's economic state had already recovered by then and the real national income per capita was back to pre-war levels by 1955 (Cabinet Office 1955). However, the economy's recovery did not stop the decline in fertility. Since then, the NRR temporarily exceeded 1 between 1967 and 1974, mainly during the second baby boom. Apart from that, fertility has almost consistently trended down (Ishikawa 2007; Beppu 2014).

In this period, fertility declined because married couples limited the number of children they had—not because the number of married individuals decreased. The marriage rate had been quite high in Japan until the 1970s. The percentage of 50-year olds who never married was less than 10 %; Japan was virtually a 'universal marriage' society. The number of children among married couples mostly ranged between one and three, with the mode being two. Given that the number of children per married couple was 3.5 in 1952, it has seen a considerable decline during the subsequent 20 years, to 2.2 children per married couple in 1972 (National Institute of Population and Social Security Research 2012).

The situation of the post-1980 fertility decline is different. Japan left the 'universal marriage' society (Kato 2011), entering the stage of the second demographic transition. Since then, the percentage 50-year olds who never married increased each year. Even when people did marry, the age at which they married increased. The fertility decline of recent years is primarily due to this reduced ability to marry.

In other words, in the cohort immediately prior to the 1960s, one adopted what is considered, even today, the 'standard' Japanese lifestyle by marrying early and building a family that consists of a husband who is the breadwinner, a full-time housewife, and two children on average. In contrast, with the 1960s cohort, a diversity of life course that did not fit in this 'standard' emerged. The timing of marriage was delayed, the number of 50-year olds who never married increased, and to continue working in order to pursue an occupational career became an acceptable option for women. In Japan, those who were single barely had children. In addition, the delay in marriage led women to postpone pregnancy, which caused an unintended drop in fertility. In these ways, changes in marital behaviour affected the decrease in fertility.

By the late 1980s, the Japanese government recognised the decline in fertility as a crisis. The level of fertility is calculated based on the simple period total fertility rate (TFR) and published every year. When this rate dropped to 1.57 (the lowest recorded rate, even lower than the previous lowest rate, recorded in 1966, due to the so-called 'year of Fire Horse superstition') in 1989, which made headlines and was called 'the 1.57 shock' (Suzuki 2013: 2). In response, various measures were implemented. However, fertility never increased and the NRR fell to 0.67 in 2010.

Women born between 1960 and 1969 were between 41 and 50 years old in 2010. They are at the age by which they have ended their reproductive period. In other words, it has now finally become possible to describe the 1960s cohort's reproduction process throughout their life course, which announced the beginning of the era of lowest fertility, the marriage decline, and the second demographic transition, which began in the 1980s and has continued to the present in Japan.

References

Aoki, Hisao. 1970. Wagakuni-no shusshoryoku-to shusshoyokusei-no tenbo (A general view of fertility and its regulation in Japan). *Jinko Mondai Kenkyu (Journal of Population Problems)* 114: 5–20 (in Japanese).

Beppu, Motomi. 2014. Zenkoku jinko-no saiseisan-ni kansuru shuyo shihyo: 2013. *Jinko Mondai Kenkyu (Journal of Population Problems)* 70(4): 512–527 (in Japanese).

Cabinet Office (Naikakufu). 1955. *Watashitachi-no Hataraki-to Kurashi: Wakariyasui Kokuminshotoku-no Hanashi (Kokuminshotoku Kaisetsu Shiryo Dai-4-go)*. Tokyo: Toyo Keizai Shinposha (in Japanese).

Hirosima, Kiyosi. 2001. Decomposing recent fertility decline: How have nuptiality and marital fertility affected it in Japan? *IUSSP seminar on "international perspectives on low fertility: Trends, theories and policies"*. Tokyo, 21–23 March 2001.

Honda, Tatsuo. 1962. 60-nendai Nihon-no jinko mondai: Sono rekishiteki jyokyo-no bunseki. *Jinkomondai Kenkyujo Nenpo* 7: 1–4 (in Japanese).

Institute for International Cooperation, Japan International Corporation Agency. 2003. *Second study on international cooperation for population and development: New insights from the Japanese experience (Executive summary)*.

Ishikawa, Akira. 2007. Zenkoku jinko-no saiseisan-ni kansuru shuyo shihyo: 2006. *Jinko Mondai Kenkyu (Journal of Population Problems)* 63(4): 74–83 (in Japanese).

Iwasawa, Miho. 2008. Shokon, rikon-no doko-to shusshoritsu-eno eikyo (Recent trends in first marriage and divorce and their effects on fertility change in Japan). *Jinko Mondai Kenkyu (Journal of Population Problems)* 64(4): 19–34 (in Japanese).

Kato, Akihiko. 2011. Mikonka-wo oshisusumetekita 2-tsuno chikara: Keizai seicho-no teika-to kojinshugi-no ideorogi (Two major factors behind the marriage decline in Japan: The deterioration in macroeconomic performance and the diffusion of individual ideology). *Jinko Mondai Kenkyu (Journal of Population Problems)* 67(2): 3–39 (in Japanese).

Mainichi Newspapers Population Problems Research Council (Mainichi Shinbun Sha Jinko Mondai Chosakai). 2000. *Nihon-no Jinko: Sengo 50-nen-no Kiseki*. Tokyo: Mainichi Shinbun Sha. Jinko Mondai Chosakai (in Japanese).

National Institute of Population and Social Security Research (IPSS) (Kokuritsu Shakai Hosho Jinko Mondai Kenkyujo). 2012. *Dai 14-kai Shussho Doko Kihon Chosa Dai-1 Hokokusho: Wagakuni Fufu-no Kekkon Katei-to Shusshoryoku (Report on the Fourteenth Japanese national fertility survey in 2010: Marriage process and fertility of married couples).* (Survey Series No. 29) (in Japanese).

Ochiai, Emiko (Translated by The Simul Press). 1997. *The Japanese family system in transition: A sociological analysis of family change in Postwar Japan (LTCB international library selection, no. 6).* Tokyo: LTCB International Library Foundation.

Okazaki, Ayanori. 1955. Nihon-ni okeru yuseiseisaku-to sono koka-nitsuite. *Jinko Mondai Kenkyu (Journal of Population Problems)* 61: 1–7 (in Japanese).

Suzuki, Toru. 2013. *Low fertility and population aging in Japan and Eastern Asia.* Tokyo: Springer.

Tachi, Mimoru. 1969. *Nippon-no Jinko Mondai* (Population problems in Japan) (Jinko Mondai Kenkyujo Kenkyu Shiryo Dai-190-go) (Institute of Population Problems Research Series No. 190) (in Japanese).

Van de Kaa, D.J. 1987. Europe's second demographic transition. *Population Bulletin* 42(1): 1–59.

Yamaguchi, Kiichi, and Akiko Yajima. 1973. Sengo-ni okeru Nihon joshi-no shusshoryoku-saisei-sanryoku-no suii (Trends in fertility and reproductivity for the Japanese female population: 1947–1972). *Jinko Mondai Kenkyu (Journal of Population Problems)* 128: 43–56 (in Japanese).

Chapter 2
Cohort Analysis of Pregnancy Attempts

Abstract The number of pregnancy attempts that do not result in live birth is estimated for the cohorts born between 1953 and 1988 (sampled every five years) based on data for age-specific fertility rates from the *Vital Statistics* of Japan and on a theoretical model of the probability of infertility and spontaneous abortions derived from the literature on medicine and demography studies. I obtain an age profile to use for estimating the probability of pregnancy attempts by women in each cohort. For women born in the 1950s, the probability of a pregnancy attempt was high in their 20s, at 20 %, and rapidly decreased in their 30s. For women born in the 1960s, the rate was 10–15 % in their 20s and rapidly decreased in their 30s. The cohort total fertility rate thus started to decline in the 1960s cohort, due to declines in marriage and a delayed social life-cycle. For women born after the 1970s, this trend has continued. Reproduction is now mainly conducted by women in their 30s. Despite the considerable increase in the number of pregnancy attempt by women older than 35 years in today's Japan, the number of childbirths has not increased, because of the increasing possibility of infertility and spontaneous abortions stemming from biological causes.

Keywords Estimated pregnancy attempt · Postponing childbirth · CTFR (cohort total fertility rate) · Abortion · Infertility

2.1 Life Course as a Sociological Perspective

A life course is defined as 'a sequence of socially defined events and roles that the individual enacts over time' (Giele and Elder 1998: 22). The life course perspective enables a holistic understanding of lives over time and across changing social contexts (Daaleman and Elder 2007). The concept of 'cohort' is a useful tool for the life course study. 'Ryder (1965) proposed the term cohort as a context for studying the life course in relation to social change. Cohort refers to the age at which people enter a social system; thus, a birth cohort locates people in history according to their year of birth' (Shanahan et al. 2003: 192). I adopt the concept

Y. Senda, *Childbearing and Careers of Japanese Women Born in the 1960s*,
Population Studies of Japan, DOI 10.1007/978-4-431-55066-2_2

of 'birth cohort' to describe and investigate how Japanese society has followed its lowest-low fertility. Hereafter, I use 'cohort' to mean 'birth cohort'.

After the 1980s, Japanese society faced lower fertility mainly due to marriage decline. This phenomenon, which was new at the time, continues even today. Japanese society still has difficulty dealing with this phenomenon, even though it recognizes that this fertility decline will have a significant impact on population structure in the future. The objective of this chapter is to review the basic situation of this fertility decline by conducting an analysis of pregnancy attempts within a cohort.

2.2 Cohort Total Fertility Rate

Cohort Total Fertility Rate (CTFR) is the index of fertility for a given generation. It is calculated by adding together the past fertility rate for each age (15–49) for the group of women who all were born in the same year (cohort). As displayed on the graph in Fig. 2.1, the bell-shaped curves indicate the age-specific fertility rate (i.e., the number of childbirths per woman of a specific age per year), and the CTFR is equal to the area between the curve and the X axis. The CTFR cannot be calculated until a given cohort reaches the age of 50, because it is only at 50 that a cohort is considered as having finished all of their reproduction processes. Therefore, TFR (the fertility rate for a given year adjusted for the age structure difference in the female population) is often used instead.

The TFR and CTFR will be the same when the fertility rate by age is the same among all cohorts. However, in reality fertility behaviour varies by cohort (Ministry of Health, Labour and Welfare 2015). TFR is convenient for forecasting, but confirmation by CTFR is necessary.

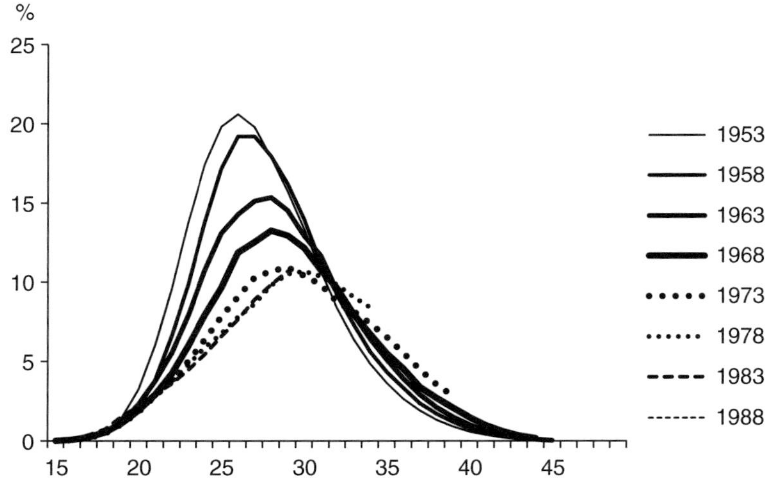

Fig. 2.1 Birth cohorts (1953–1988) and the age-specific fertility rate (%). *Source Data Vital Statistics*, 1968–2012

In Japan, the CTFR fell sharply in the 1960s cohort: as can be seen in Fig. 2.1, the lines for '1963' and '1968' are at lower positions than those for '1953' and '1958'. Why did the CTFR fall so sharply in the 1960s cohort? This book aims to examine the cause from the perspective of the relationship between women's fertility behaviours and their employment behaviours.

2.3 Trends in the Fertility Rate by Age and by Birth Cohort

We will begin by looking at the overall situation of fertility decline in Fig. 2.1. The graph shows the fertility rate at each age among women who were born between 1953 and 1988. The observation ends in 2012 because that is the most recently available data on the number of births. In the following analysis, the data used for the estimates is grouped in five-year increments: 20–24, 25–29, etc. to 45–49. Therefore, it is sufficient for the upper age of the age groups by five-year increment hits the year 2012 (i.e., this allows the data to be analysed all the way to 2012). Specifically, it is ideal to analyse the cohorts that consist of individuals who were born in a year with the last digit of '3' or '8'. For example, since $2012 - 1968 = 44$, analysing the 1968 cohort will allow us to use the data for the 40–44 years old.

Likewise, since $2012 - 1963 = 49$, analysing the 1963 cohort will allow us to use the data for 45–49 years old.

The highest fertility rate for the 1953 cohort was 20.6 %, which was observed in 1976, when members of the cohort were 26 years old. This value fell to 2.6 % at when the members of the cohort reached age 36. For the most part, this cohort completes their reproduction process in their early 30s.

For the subsequent cohorts, fertility during their 20s declined. According to Fig. 2.1, the greatest decline in fertility among those in their 20s occurred between the 1958 and 1963 cohorts. Fertility among those in their 20s continued to fall afterwards; however, it stopped its decline in the 1973 cohort, as well as in later cohorts.

Compared to the considerable fertility decline that began in the early years among those in their 20s, the change in births among those in their 30s occurred more slowly. Although the 1963 and 1968 cohorts' fertility during their 20s was significantly lower compared to the 1950s cohort, their fertility in their 30s was almost the same as that of the 1950s cohort.

Births given among those in their 30s or older began to increase in the later cohorts. Compared to prior cohorts, childbirths up to the age of 39 (in 2012) increased in the 1973 cohort, shifting the fertility rate curve to the right. In the 1978 cohort (the data is available only for those up to 34 years old), the drop in the fertility rate between their late 20s and early 30s was much smaller than that of the prior cohorts (i.e., they continued the reproduction process into their 30s). Although the fertility rate of its members in their 20s fell considerably in the 1970s cohort, the reproduction process continued into their 30s, while their fertility rate in their late 30s increased.

If the increase in their fertility rate in their 30s was large enough to offset the decrease in the fertility rate in their 20s, it only means that the timing of childbirth shifted from the 20s to 30s, and that the CTFR would not be lower when compared to the previous rate. However, the increase in births by women in their 30s or older among those in the 1963 and later cohorts was not enough to compensate for the fertility decline they experienced in their 20s. Overall fertility, therefore, continues to trend down in the younger cohorts (Moriizumi 2007).

2.4 Analytical Perspective of This Chapter

The most popular model for the theoretical explanation of this phenomenon is that the timing of childbirth and the number of children in a family are determined by the rational decisions of the involved parties (Ohbuchi et al. 1998; Takayama et al. 2000). The woman's (or couple's) intentions and plans for childbirth are certainly important in making a decision about giving birth; this is confirmed by the data analyses of Yamaguchi (2004, 2009) and Senda (2007). Japan's central government and local governments also use this kind of model to design countermeasures to the falling fertility rate. 'Reforming the way of work based on the keyword 'work-life balance'', 'expanding childcare services in the local community', and 'providing economic support to families that are raising children' are the three pillars of one such policy (Moriizumi 2010; Kamata 2010). All three pillars are based on the idea that the woman herself, or the couple, rationally make a decision regarding childbirth.

However, the 'outcome' of whether to give birth sometimes does not coincide with the intention of the parties. Iwasawa (2002) used data from the *11th National Fertility Survey* (1997) to analyse fertility intentions for additional births. She calculated the incidence of various combinations of intentions and outcomes. The results indicated the following: (1) a substantial proportion of births in contemporary Japan are unintended ones (i.e., the cases of births where the parents did not want a child or wanted a child later), and (2) there are also a considerable number of cases that do not lead to birth despite the parents' intention for additional births. These results demonstrate that the probability of a pregnancy attempt leading to an actual pregnancy, and then to childbirth, is an important factor in determining fertility, as well as whether a pregnancy attempt is made by a woman and man.

When the time frame for having children is delayed, these unintended fertility determinants become more important. This is because it is empirically known that the probability of pregnancy declines as the woman and man age, and the probability of spontaneous abortion and the risks in pregnancy and childbirth also increase for the mother. These issues were not so critical in the past because most women used to give birth in their 20s, as seen in Fig. 2.1. Then, the difference between the number of births and the parents' attempts to have children was not so large as to be a problem. In other words, the model in which couples rationally make decisions regarding whether to have a child was able to explain fertility. The fertility behaviour of the 1950s cohort can be explained by the 'rational decision-making of the parties' model.

However, the early 30s age groups have the largest number of births since 2005 (*Vital Statistics*). The number of women who give birth in their late 30s has begun to increase. Those who gave birth in their 40s or later also increased. In this way, the increase in births at an age when the probability of pregnancy declines, and the probability of spontaneous abortion rises, shows that we cannot ignore the number of deliberate attempts in which parents want a child that do not lead to birth. It is becoming apparent that the model in which couples make rational decisions faces limitations in explaining fertility, making it necessary to conduct a new analysis in order to estimate the extent to which pregnancy attempts are made.

The fertility behaviour of the 1960s and later cohorts must be analysed based on the perspective of how often unexpected, unintended, and disappointing events occur for parties who cannot have children even though they want to.

This chapter will estimate the number of pregnancy attempts from the observed number of live births. Birth is a phenomenon that occurs as a result of sexual intercourse or artificial insemination; however, these acts do not always lead to fertility. There should be a considerable number of cases that do not result in a birth due to infertility, spontaneous abortion, induced abortion, stillbirth, etc. There is very little understanding in modern Japanese society as to how many cases that do not result in births exist. This is quite a contrast to the accurate understanding of the number of cases that resulted in birth in the *Vital Statistics* compiled by the Ministry of Health, Labour, and Welfare.

In what follows, a rough estimate for cases that do not result in a birth will be tried, using the knowledge of existing medical and population sciences. Data on maternal age will be used, since the probabilities of infertility and spontaneous abortion vary greatly by age. There have been many studies on this subject, which will utilise in this chapter. As a note, Senda (2011) used data on the number of births per year by mother's age to analyse changes in pregnancy attempts in a cross-sectional term. The analysis in this chapter organises the data in terms of cohort and applies the same method as Senda (2011).

2.5 Pregnancy Attempts

Since birth in modern society occurs as a result of individual decisions, the intention of the parties is extremely important. The intentions for giving birth can be divided into two types. The first is the number of children (quantity) compared to how many (additional) children the parents wish to have. The second is the timing of when to have children. Iwasawa and Mita (2007) analysed the *National Fertility Survey* data, demonstrating the following: (1) the number of women who try to have additional children in their 30s and older is increasing, and (2) the preferred timing varies among these women, because some want children as soon as possible while others want children after a while or do not have any specific idea. Unfortunately, this study did not analyse whether those who wanted children as soon as possible took any action to make pregnancy possible or, conversely, whether those who did not wish to have children refrained from behaviours that might make them pregnant.

Unlike studies on intention, this study estimates behaviours that are directly related to pregnancy. The term 'pregnancy attempt', defined as 'any intentional action that might lead to pregnancy' was employed. It typically means having a sexual intercourse without contraception. However, the concept also covers a wider spectrum, including cases involving a passive intention, such as 'I don't mind getting pregnant'; more proactive cases in which the individual is thinking 'I want to have a child as soon as possible'; and cases in which the individual undergoes fertility treatment at obstetrics and gynaecology facilities or uses assisted reproductive technologies, such as in vitro fertilisation. The concept of a 'pregnancy attempt' (Basso et al. 2000) is appropriate for representing these behaviours.

Even if an individual does intentionally engage in behaviour that might result in pregnancy, it does not always result in a birth. Cases of pregnancy attempts that do not result in a birth could include: (1) cases in which the woman does not become pregnant (fecundity issue), (2) cases in which the woman becomes pregnant but ends up having a spontaneous abortion or stillbirth, and (3) cases in which the woman voluntarily undergoes induced abortion (Wood 1994). Of these factors, fecundity is known to decline with age. Furthermore, the probability of spontaneous abortion increases with age. Either way, the effect of advancing age on pregnancy is an important factor affecting the gap between pregnancy attempts and births. Heffner (2004) and the Research Group for Women and the Declining Birth Rate (2005) used the data of Andersen et al. (2000) and Menken et al. (1986) to present methods for decomposing these factors. This chapter follows these methods in order to construct estimates regarding pregnancy attempts that did not result in a birth.

Unfortunately, the collected data on induced abortions, infertility, and spontaneous abortions found in the current Japanese statistical system are inadequate. Therefore, this chapter will use available data sources, such as Danish medical statistic data (Andersen et al. 2000) and international research data on natural fertility (Menken et al. 1986). Due to this limitation, my estimation will be very simple and rough.

2.6 Pregnancy Attempts that Do not Result in a Birth

As seen above, the cases of pregnancy attempts that do not result in a birth include the following: (1) induced abortion, (2) stillbirth and spontaneous abortion, and (3) infertility. In the following section, we will examine how frequently these cases occur in contemporary Japan.

2.6.1 Induced Abortion

In Japan, the number of induced abortions is published every year by the *Eugenic Protection Statistics*, *Maternal Body Protection Statistics* and the *Report on Public*

Health Administration and Services by MHLW, which aggregates the reports that physicians file with prefectures upon performing an induced abortion.

Here we summarise these statistics according to Senda (2011). In 1955, the statistics included 1,169,079 induced abortions and 1,730,689 births. The ratio was about 2:3. This ratio declined to about 1:3 in 1970, and remained at that level until 1990. Then, it further declined to about 1:5 in 2009 (223,388 induced abortions to 1,070,029 births). Thus, induced abortions in Japanese society dramatically decreased in the past half-century, in terms of both number and ratio (Senda 2011).

That being said, a significant number of induced abortions are still being performed even today. In addition, the ratio of induced abortions to the number of births varies across age groups. The lowest ratio is observed among those in their early 30s, while higher ratios are seen among the younger and older groups. Based on the 2009 data, whereas the ratio for those in their early 30s was about 1:10, it rose to 1:5 and 1:2 for those in their late 30s and those in their 40s, respectively.

Therefore, a considerable number of induced abortions are performed even today, especially within the older age group. For this chapter, which focuses on pregnancy at an older age, induced abortion is a factor that should definitely be taken into account. However, there are probably cases of induced abortions that were performed because the pregnancy was unintended or unwanted, or because there was no choice but to terminate it even though it was attempted.[1] While the latter is a subject of discussion for this chapter, which covers the gap between pregnancy attempts and births, the former is not. However, we cannot distinguish between these two types using the currently available data. Therefore, this chapter will only point out the large number of induced abortions without conducting any further examination.

2.6.2 Stillbirth and Spontaneous Abortion

Next, we will examine those terminations of pregnancy that do not result from artificial treatment. *Vital Statistics* aggregates non-artificial pregnancy terminations that occur at the 12th week of pregnancy or later as ‘natural stillbirth’. The number of natural stillbirths is about 1 % of the number of births. When looking at this by age, although the figure increases among those in their late 40s, it still remains at about 5 % (Senda 2011). Therefore, it will not have a significant impact, even if we ignore the cases that fall under this category.

In contrast, it is believed that there is a very large number of so-called ‘early abortions’, which refer to a termination of pregnancy at less than 12 weeks of pregnancy (Suzumori 2004: 318). However, these cases are not captured in the *Vital Statistics* or in any clinical database in Japan. It is therefore difficult to obtain accurate data.

---

[1]Pregnancy in old age increases the probability of chromosome abnormality. It seems that there are many cases in which an induced abortion is chosen for this reason, because the technologies to prenatally predict and diagnose such cases have advanced in recent years (Yoshimizu 2006).

The *National Fertility Survey*, published by the National Institute of Population and Social Security Research (IPSS), provides a clue for solving this issue. It includes a question that asks about recipients' experiences, including spontaneous abortion, that relate to the subject's history of pregnancy and childbirth (Sato and Iwasawa 1998). Table 2.1 shows the results tabulated from the *14th National Fertility Survey* in 2010 on up to five pregnancies experienced by the women recipients (IPSS 2012: 131–134). The survey did not differentiate stillbirths and spontaneous abortions; these are shown together under the category of 'stillbirth and spontaneous abortion' in Table 2.1. As mentioned above, the majority of incidents in this category might consist of spontaneous abortions during early pregnancy.

We can see from Table 2.1 that the probability of a stillbirth or spontaneous abortion increases as the age at the time of pregnancy increases. The ratio of the number of stillbirths and spontaneous abortions to the number of live births (a/b) found in the right column of Table 2.1 is below 1:9 among pregnancies for all of the ages up to around 30. In comparison, the ratio for pregnancies in the mid-30s is about 1:5, and increases to more than 1:3 for pregnancies among women in their late 30s or later.

However, this data could have a large margin of error. The number of responses from pregnant women 35 or older is small. The sampling error might therefore large. Furthermore, another possible source of error is the bias stemming from the possibility that past negative experiences are less likely to be reported because

Table 2.1 Frequency of stillbirths and spontaneous abortions by women's history of pregnancy and childbirth

Age at pregnancy	Live birth (b)	Stillbirth and spontaneous abortion (a)	a/b
–14	0	0	–
15–18	78	6	0.077
19–20	307	26	0.085
21–22	622	47	0.076
23–24	1267	99	0.078
25–26	1826	190	0.104
27–28	2130	220	0.103
29–30	1870	204	0.109
31–32	1322	182	0.138
33–34	867	141	0.163
35–36	433	81	0.187
37–38	198	61	0.308
39–40	59	37	0.627
41–42	18	8	0.444
43–44	3	5	1.667
Unknown	222	73	0.329

Data The 2010 14th National Fertility Survey questionnaire for couples (IPSS 2012: 214–218). The total figures for the first to fifth pregnancies are based on the question on pregnancy experience (Q12). The responses to 'birth and spontaneous abortion (including stillbirth) regarding your pregnancy' are tabulated

the survey uses a distributed and self-administered questionnaire to ask women to answer retrospectively about their pregnancy and childbirth history.

Therefore, in order to find more reliable data for estimating the probability of incidences such as spontaneous abortion, The Danish data provided in Andersen et al. (2000), which used the civil registration system in Denmark, will be used. Andersen et al. (2000) collected data on all pregnancy results between 1978 and 1992 by using personal identification to merge the data that hospitals are required to report—such as stillbirths, spontaneous abortions, and induced abortions—with data on a woman's history of childbirth. The data on stillbirths and spontaneous abortions are from the National Discharge Registry, which was created based on the hospitals' diagnoses.

Supposing that there are not many social or cultural factors related to the causes of spontaneous abortions in Japan, the probability of spontaneous abortion at each age should not differ much. To be sure, this point is different from the situation in Japan, since women in Denmark can terminate pregnancy up to the 12th week of pregnancy at public hospitals, free of charge, for any reason whatsoever (Knudsen 1999). In addition, since the number of spontaneous abortions is counted based on the definition 'it is a termination prior to the 29th week of pregnancy', this is different from the cut-off for spontaneous abortion in obstetrics in Japan (which occurs at less than 22 weeks of pregnancy). Keeping those differences in mind, we will continue to examine the Danish data.

The number of pregnancies that did not result in a live birth was estimated using the Danish data (Table 2.2). Here I count stillbirths (s), spontaneous abortions (a), and ectopic pregnancies (e). The ratio was calculated against the number of live births (b), as shown in the (a + e + s)/b column in Table 2.2.

Table 2.2 Number of stillbirths and spontaneous abortions by the age of women based on the Danish data (1978–1992)

Age	Live birth (b)	Spontaneous abortion (a)	Ectopic pregnancy (e)	Stillbirth (s)	Total (p)	(a + e + s)/b	(a + s)/b	b/p
12–19	44,674	5427	808	223	51,132	0.145	0.126	0.874
20–24	246,038	24,465	4163	1046	275,712	0.121	0.104	0.892
25–29	312,904	33,728	7233	1270	355,135	0.135	0.112	0.881
30–34	157,457	22,391	5861	699	186,408	0.184	0.147	0.845
35–39	43,471	11,369	2679	226	57,745	0.328	0.267	0.753
40–44	5101	3962	614	34	9711	0.904	0.783	0.525
45–	117	509	54	1	681	4.821	4.359	0.172
Total of pregnancies	809,762	101,851	21,412	3499	936,524	0.157	0.130	0.865
Total of persons	509,867	85,838	18,968	3457	618,130	0.212	0.175	0.825

Source Civil Registration System; National Discharge Registry (Andersen et al. 2000: 1709)
Hydatidiform moles and deliveries of stillborn child that are less than 29 weeks are considered spontaneous abortions. Those that occur afterwards are considered stillbirths

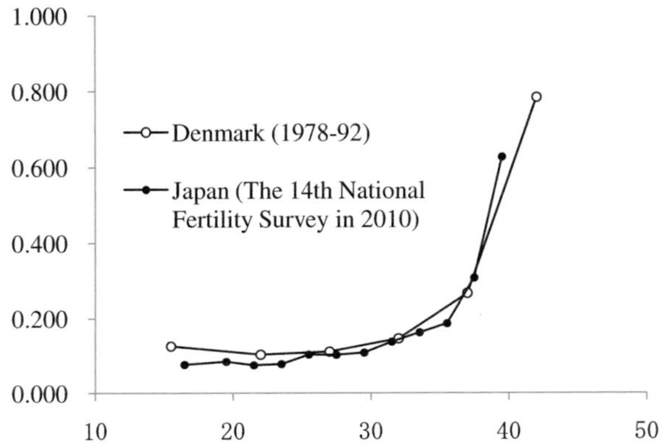

Fig. 2.2 Incident rate of stillbirths and spontaneous abortions by women's age. The values for Japan were calculated as a/b from Table 2.1, while the figures for Denmark were calculated by (a + s)/b from Table 2.2. The horizontal axis shows the midpoint for each age classification (the Danish data for those 45 or older and Japanese data for those 41 or older are excluded)

Although the ratio between the number of births and the number of spontaneous abortions is about 1:10 among those in their early 20s, it increases as age increases; we can see that it reaches 1:3 and 9:10 in their late 30s and early 40s, respectively. Andersen et al. (2000) checked the effects of such factors as the woman's birth cohort, the calendar year of pregnancy, and whether the woman is multiparous. They found that these factors do affect the risk for spontaneous abortion, but the differences due to these factors are within a few percent of each other. They accordingly concluded that the patterns of the ratio of spontaneous abortion by age are the same when the effects of these factors are controlled.

Figure 2.2 compares the data on stillbirth and spontaneous abortion in Japan (Table 2.1) and Denmark (Table 2.2). Since the *National Fertility Survey* in Japan allows for the respondent to determine what spontaneous abortion is, it is possible that ectopic pregnancy is not regarded as spontaneous abortion (or not recognised as pregnancy). Therefore, when preparing Fig. 2.2, I calculated (a + s)/b by excluding ectopic pregnancy from the data for Denmark. The patterns by age are similar in both Japan and Denmark. Although there are small differences (the line for the Japanese data is slightly below that of Denmark), it seems fine to assume that the basic pattern of stillbirth and spontaneous abortion by age is also similar between Japan and Denmark.

2.6.3 Infertility

In addition to stillbirths, induced abortions, and spontaneous abortions, infertility is also a factor that can result in pregnancy attempts that do not lead to a birth.

The Japan Society of Obstetrics and Gynaecology (JSOG 2008: 276) defines 'infertility' or 'sterility' as 'a case in which the male and female in their reproductive years do not become pregnant even though they wish to and stay sexually active without contraception for a period of time'. Although it is said that about 10 % of all married couples are infertile (Hoshi 2004), there is no scientific evidence for this figure (Senba 2003: 76), or any reliable statistics. The number of patients being treated at hospitals for infertility is only partially tracked, and it is also not clear as to how many infertile individuals do not go to the hospital (Oishi 2007). Therefore, it is difficult to know the exact number of infertility incidences.

The probability of infertility increases in old age (Wood 1994: 37). Therefore, incidences of infertility are important data when dealing with a decline in fertility due to a delayed reproduction process. However, we are not concerned with an understanding of the incidence of infertility itself. All that is necessary is the ability to estimate the overall number of pregnancy attempts that do not result in a birth while taking infertility and all other factors into consideration.

As described above, the main reasons for pregnancy attempts that do not result in births are infertility and spontaneous abortion, if induced abortion is not considered. Meanwhile, of the cases that do not result in a birth even though the egg is fertilised, only those cases of confirmed pregnancy are recognised as spontaneous abortion. Infertility probably includes cases in which the woman is actually pregnant but not clinically confirmed (Ozawa et al. 2010). If you think of it this way, it is not meaningful to try to distinguish between infertility and spontaneous abortion. As described below, the number of pregnancy attempts that do not result in births will be directly estimated, including both of infertility and spontaneous abortion.

2.7 Estimating Pregnancy Attempts

In what follows, the research results of Menken et al. (1986) will be referred to, which applied the research data on natural fertility produced by Henry (1961) in order to estimate the number of pregnancy attempts that do not result in a birth. Their study provides an estimated effect of couples' ages on fertility for a population of couples who are not consciously controlling for their number of children (Menken and Larsen 1986). The study results report that, although the overall level of fertility is quite different among populations, the effect of a woman's age can be observed across the board. Using the early 20s as the baseline, fertility declines by 6 % for women in their late 20s, 14 % for those in their early 30s, 31 % in their late 30s, 64 % in their early 40s, and 95 % in their late 40s (Menken and Larsen 1986: 152; Menken et al. 1986: 1389). Please note that, although the age of men might also determine fertility (De La Rochebrochard and Thonneau 2002; Dunson et al. 2002), only the age of women will be addressed in the discussion below.

Using these values and the number of births, how many pregnancy attempts exist by cohort during the reproduction process will be calculated, as shown in Fig. 2.1. In the following estimate, I assumed that infertility is not present (i.e., there is only the risk of spontaneous abortion) in the baseline population (those in their early 20s). In other words, the probability that a pregnancy attempt will result in a birth for those in their early 20s is set at 0.892, based on the value in the far right column b/p of Table 2.2. Likewise, the probability that the pregnancy attempt will result in a birth among those in their teens is 0.874, assuming that they only face the risk of spontaneous abortion. For those in their late 20s, I assumed a 6 % decline from the baseline, in accordance with Menken and Larsen (1986) and set it as $0.892 \times 0.94 = 0.838$. Those in their 30s and 40s were handled in a similar way: the birth rate for those in their early 30s is $0.892 \times 0.86 = 0.767$, for those in their late 30s it is $0.892 \times 0.69 = 0.615$, for the early 40s it is $0.892 \times 0.36 = 0.321$, and for the late 40s it is $0.892 \times 0.05 = 0.045$. For women age 50 or older, I assume the rate is the same as for those in their late 40s, 0.045. Although the data on the number of births is available in one-year increments, I grouped them in five-year increments to estimate the number of pregnancy attempts using the above theoretical ratio. The estimated results are shown in Fig. 2.3.

The data for those in their 20s do not differ so much from those presented in Fig. 2.1. In other words, the 1953 cohort reaches its highest peak when its members are in their late 20s. The number of births gradually declines for subsequent cohorts. In the past, many pregnancy attempts took place while women were still quite young, in their 20s. Since there is hardly any infertility or spontaneous abortion present in this age group, the fertility rate reached a high level (the probability of pregnancy attempts resulting in a birth was high). However, this number had significantly dropped in the 1963 cohort and has continued falling since then.

Regarding the birth rate for those in their 30s, there is no significant difference between Figs. 2.1 and 2.3, at least up to the 1960s cohort. For these cohorts, the number of pregnancy attempts sharply declined when women reach their 30s, regardless

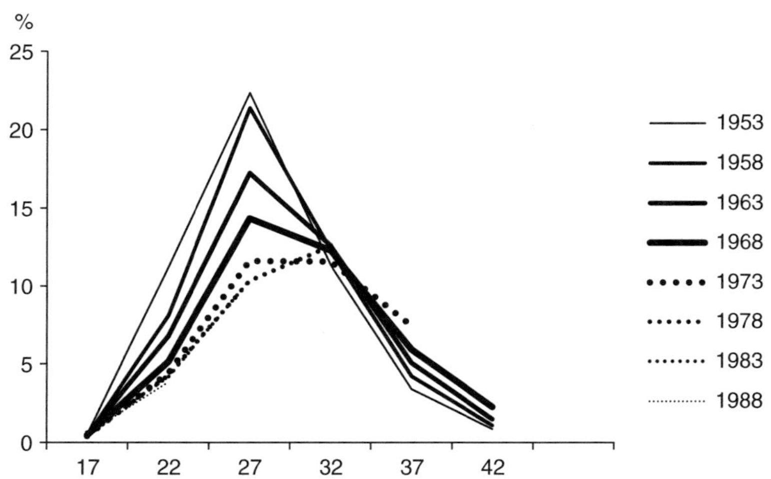

Fig. 2.3 Pregnancy attempts by birth cohort (1953–1988) and age (5-year classification)

of whether they were born in the 1950s or 1960s. Women born in the 1950s, who had attempted pregnancy with a high probability in their mid-20s, completed their reproduction process while in their 20s and demonstrate a low pregnancy rate in their 30s. Meanwhile, with those who were born in the 1960s, reproductive activity in their 30s is as inactive as for those born in the 1950s. The women in the 1960s cohort, whose pregnancy attempts were infrequent in their 20s, did not catch up in their 30s.

The cohorts from the 1970s and later demonstrate a different trend. Although the number of pregnancy attempts is even smaller for women in their 20s in the 1973 cohort, when compared to the 1968 cohort, it does not decline too much for women in their early 30s, and is maintained at a certain level even into their late 30s. With the 1978 cohort, the number of pregnancy attempts is actually higher for women in their early 30s than for those in their late 20s. In this way, those women who were born in the 1970s or later were liberated from the traditional pattern, in which pregnancy attempts dramatically fall once they reach their 30s. Women in the 1970s cohort tried to have children after they reached their 30s. However, whether they face challenges in having those children is another problem.

2.8 Changes in Social Life-Cycle and the Cohort Effect

It is plausible to say that the changes in the reproduction process among the 1950s, 1960s, and 1970s cohorts that are examined in this chapter represent the process through which Japan became a low-fertility society. This process keeps pace with changes in the social life-cycle.[2]

Refer to Figs. 2.4, 2.5, 2.6, 2.7, 2.8, 2.9 and 2.10, the cumulative frequency of births and estimated birth attempts in each cohort, respectively. Between 1953 and 1958 (Figs. 2.4 and 2.5), the curve for the cumulative frequency of births sharply rises for ages 24–29, slows down for 29–34, and remains at the same level for ages 34 and older.

Between 1963 and 1968 (Figs. 2.6 and 2.7), the sharp increase previously seen for ages 24–29 disappears, as more people remain unmarried at these ages. The frequency of births also declines. The curve of the cumulative frequency remains at the same level for the cohorts for age 34 and older.

The curve for the 1973 cohort reveals a new pattern (Fig. 2.8). An increase continues even to ages 34–39, while the rise becomes shallower than for the earlier years, during ages 24–34. Regarding the 1978 and 1983 cohorts (Figs. 2.9 and 2.10), there are not enough data at this time. However, they seem to show a similar tendency to the 1973 cohort. For the women in the 1970s cohort, the delay in the timing of pregnancy attempts brought about an increase of pregnancies in their late-30s. Note that the area between the lines for 'Attempt' and 'Birth' represents the cumulative gap between attempts and outcomes. Its size depends on the timing of the pregnancy attempts. The later the attempt, the larger this area is.

[2]The 'social life-cycle' is marked by life events such as 'changes in marital, job, and economic status index' (Scheid and Brown 2009).

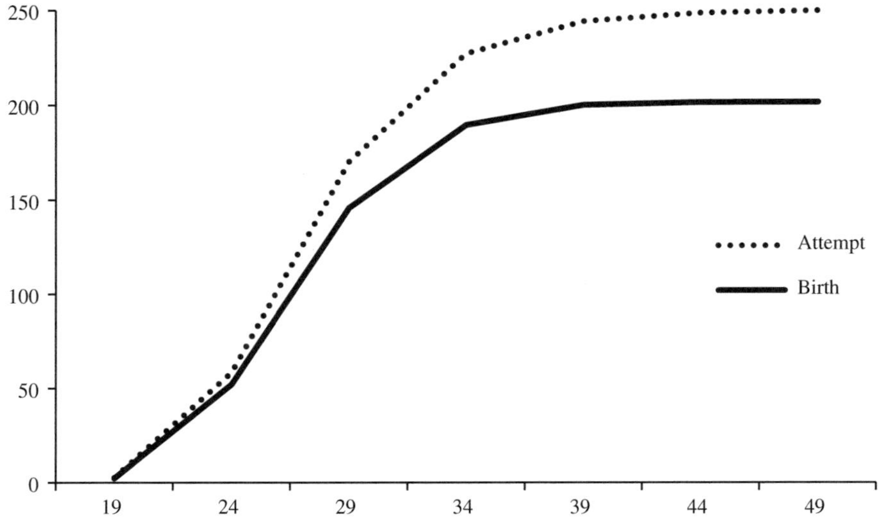

Fig. 2.4 Cumulative frequency of births and estimated birth attempts: 1953

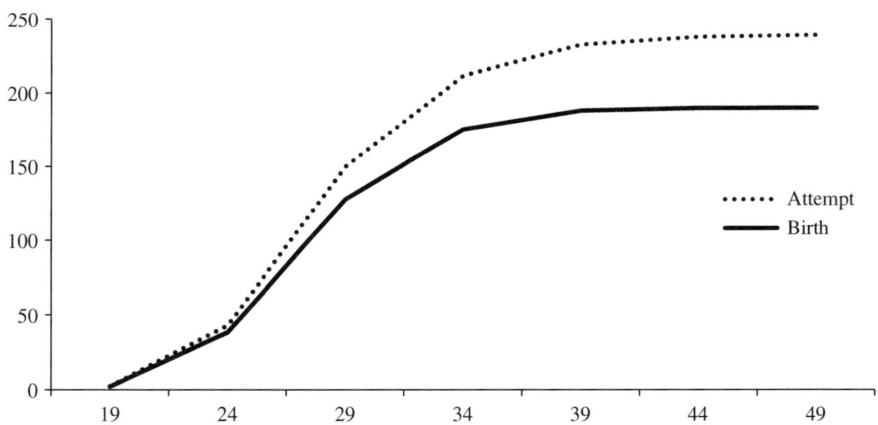

Fig. 2.5 Cumulative frequency of births and estimated birth attempts: 1958

The life course in which a woman marries and has children in her mid-20s was well established within the 1950s cohort. The reproduction process was compressed into the women's 20s; it was a common lifestyle to marry early in life and have, on average, two children.

The subsequent 1960s cohort experienced the collapse of the social life-cycle in which a woman married and had children during her 20s. Late marriages and marriage decline continued, and the choice to not marry rapidly became common in this cohort. Even if they did marry, the timing gradually shifted to later in their lives. However, the normative life-cycle, in which a woman finished having

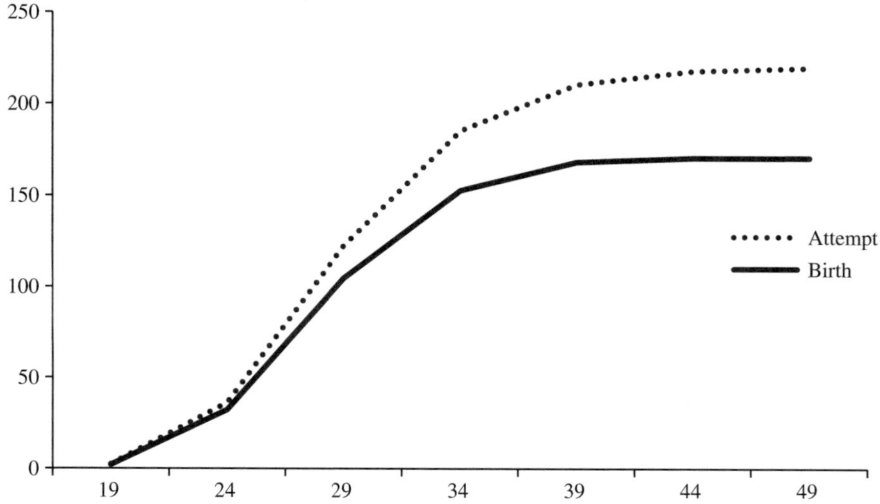

Fig. 2.6 Cumulative frequency of births and estimated birth attempts: 1963

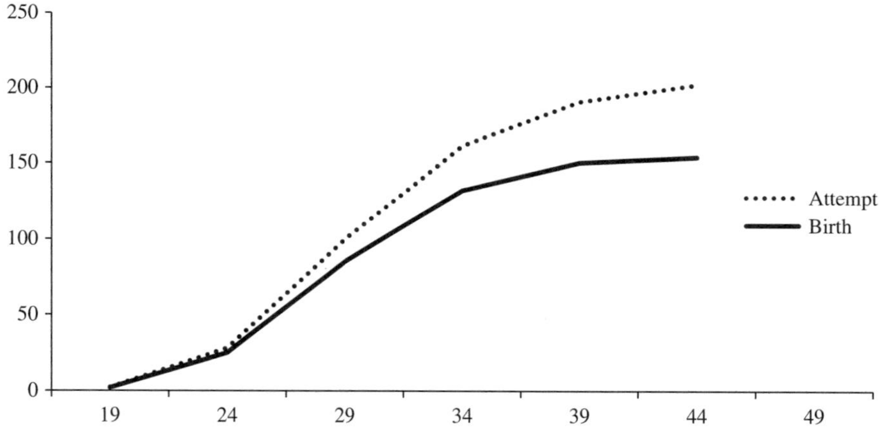

Fig. 2.7 Cumulative frequency of births and estimated birth attempts: 1968

children while in her 20s, was maintained by this cohort. Referring to Figs. 2.6 and 2.7, pregnancy attempts for the 1960s cohort were concentrated among women in their 20s, and rapidly decreased as they reached their 30s. They never recovered from the delay in the birth process in their 20s after reaching their 30s.

In contrast, women in the 1970s cohort clearly transformed the social life-cycle during their 30s. As can be seen in Fig. 2.8, the reproduction process is no longer an activity limited to one's 20s. The data in this figure exhibit the emergence of a new social life-cycle, in which women have children in their late 30s. Pregnancy has actually become something that is actively attempted after a woman reaches her 30s.

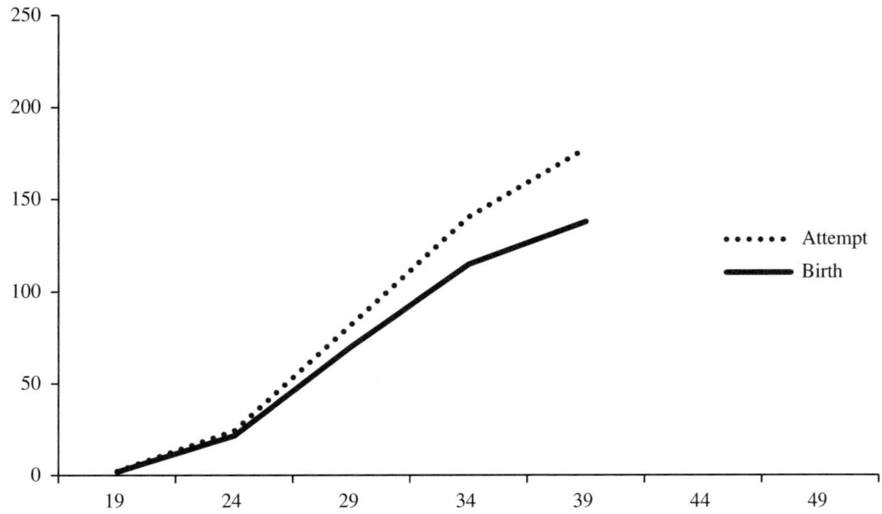

Fig. 2.8 Cumulative frequency of births and estimated birth attempts: 1973

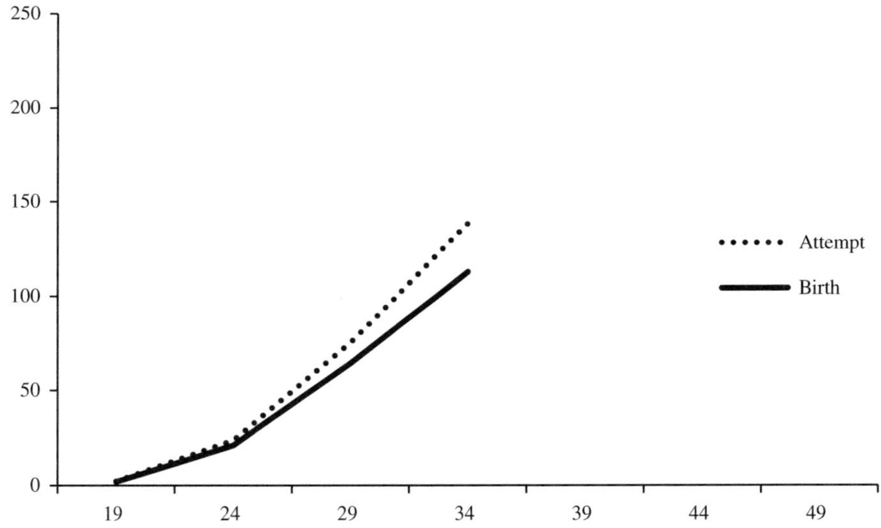

Fig. 2.9 Cumulative frequency of births and estimated birth attempts: 1978

Note that there is some uncertainty present in the data for the 1970s and subsequent cohorts, since they are in their 40s, or younger, and have therefore not yet completed their reproduction process. So, the final conclusion cannot be known until some time passes. However, if the current trend continues in its current state, we can expect the timing of the reproduction period to shift further into old age.

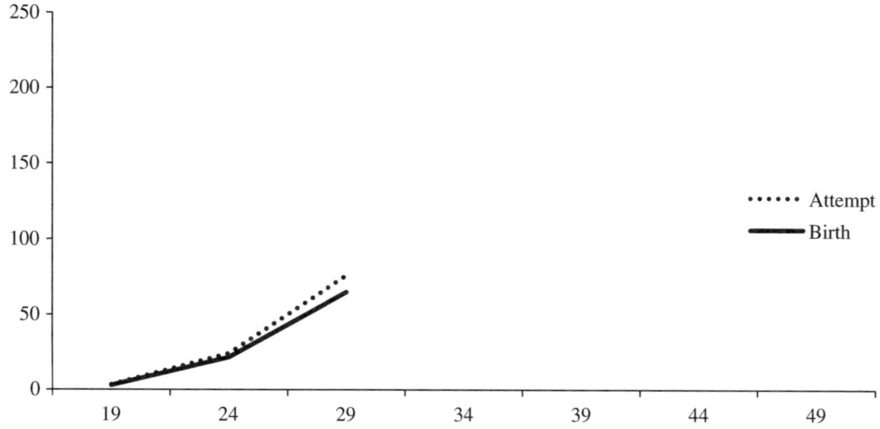

Fig. 2.10 Cumulative frequency of births and estimated birth attempts: 1983

The primary period for the reproductive process is expected to shift from a women's 20s to late-30s or later among the younger cohorts of the future.[3]

On the other hand, the possibility of pregnancy and childbirth is determined by the biological reproductive period. It is not possible for a woman to have children, even if she wanted to, if her body is not in a condition suitable to making it possible. The period in which a woman can become pregnant and give birth has not been extended too much today, even with advanced medicine.

For this reason, pregnancy attempts that do not result in a birth will increase when a woman's social life-cycle is pushed back due to changing social conditions. If a woman attempts to become pregnant is in her mid-20s, she would have about ten years before she reaches her mid-30s, when her fecundity significantly drops and the probability for spontaneous abortion increases. It is probably quite feasible to have two to three children in this period. Because of the strong norm of universal and timely marriage, this type of life course had been maintained as a standard through the 1950s cohort. Today, however, this social life-cycle has shifted to later in life. Among the 1970s and later cohorts, the probability for successfully giving birth has already decreased by the time the majority of women begin attempting pregnancy in their 30 s. Even if a woman wished to have three children, it is quite impossible that she will accomplish it by her biological time limit. Indeed, Senda (2014) estimated that 29.5 % of pregnancy attempts in 2012 did not to result in live birth, a 9-point increase from the 1985 figure of 20.4 % (Table 2.3).

[3]Billari et al. (2011) analysed surveys conducted in 25 European countries and noted that the responses to the question for the age at which a woman cannot bear a child tend to be 35, 40, 45, and 50 years old. Among them, the vast majority answered '40 years old', accounting for 40 %. This probably has to do with the fact that people tend to plan their life in five-year increments. This is important in terms of the issues regarding formation and change in social life-cycles.

Table 2.3 Trend of the estimated pregnancy attempts that do not result in births

	1955	1985	2012
Pregnancy attempts	2,229,874	1,792,413	1,468,756
Pregnancy attempts that do not result in births	499,185	360,874	431,661
Percentage of the pregnancy attempts that do not result in births (%)	22.4	20.1	29.4

This trend continues today. The Ministry of Health, Labour and Welfare also reported age-specific fertility for women in their 30s has increased, while for women in their 20s it has decreased, with the total for all ages (TFR) having slightly increased since 2006 (MLHW 2015). In recent years, looking for a marriage partner (*kon-katsu*) and methods to improve the chance of becoming pregnant (*nin-katsu*) have attracted social attention (Saito and Shirakawa 2012). However, unless there is a ground-breaking advancement in medicine that overcomes the biological limit, the number of births among those in their late 30s and older is unlikely to increase dramatically (Balasch and Gratacós 2012).

The 1960s cohort was present in the middle stage of this social change. While the number of pregnancy attempts drastically decreased among women in their 20s, it did not increase among women in their 30s. It may be that the decline in pregnancy attempts was due to delays in the timing of when to have children. However, they did not try to return to overall levels by giving birth after reaching their 30s. The 1960s cohort was thus very inactive in terms of reproduction throughout their life course. I can conclude that they ran out of time: they postponed having children in their 20s to account for their delayed social life-cycle, and then gave up childbirth once they passed the age deemed ideal by the norms of their time.

References

Andersen, Anne-Marie Nybo, Jan Wohlfahrt, Peter Christens, Jørn Olsen, and Mads Melbye. 2000. Maternal age and fetal loss: Population based register linkage study. *British Medical Journal* 320: 1708–1712.

Balasch, Juan, and Edgard Gratacós. 2012. Delayed childbearing: Effects on fertility and the outcome of pregnancy. *Current Opinion in Obstetrics and Gynecology* 24(3): 187–193.

Basso, Olga, Svend Juul, and Jørn Olsen. 2000. Time to pregnancy as a correlate of fecundity: Differential persistence in trying to become pregnant as a source of bias. *International Journal of Epidemiology* 29: 856–861.

Billari, Francesco C., Alice Goisis, Aart C. Liefbroer, Richard A. Settersten, Arnstein Aassve, Gunhild Hagestad, and Zsolt Spéder. 2011. Social age deadlines for the childbearing of women and men. *Human Reproduction* 26(3): 616–622.

Daaleman, Timothy P., and Glen H. Elder. 2007. Family medicine and the life course paradigm. *Journal of the American Board of Family Medicine* 20(1): 85–92.

De La Rochebrochard, Elise, and Patrick Thonneau. 2002. Paternal age and maternal age are risk factors for miscarriage: Results of a multicentre European study. *Human Reproduction* 17(6): 1649–1656.

Dunson, David B., Bernardo Colombo, and Donna D. Baird. 2002. Changes with age in the level and duration of fertility in the menstrual cycle. *Human Reproduction* 17(5): 1399–1403.

Giele, Janet Z., and Glen H. Elder Jr. 1998. *Methods of life course research: Qualitative and quantitative approaches*. Thousand Oaks: Sage Publications.

Heffner, Linda J. 2004. Advanced maternal age: How old is too old? *New England Journal of Medicine* 351: 1927–1929.

Henry, Louis. 1961. Some data on natural fertility. *Eugenics Quarterly* 8(2): 81–91.

Hoshi, Kazuhiko. 2004. Funin. In *Hyojun Sanka Fujinkagaku*, 3rd ed, ed. Takeshi Maruo, and Takashi Okai, 63–83. Tokyo: Igaku-Shoin (in Japanese).

Iwasawa, Miho. 2002. Kin'nen-no KikanTFR hendo-ni okeru kekkonkodo oyobi fufu-no shusshokodo-no henka-no kiyo-nitsuite (On the contribution of the changes in the first marriage behavior to the recent change in total fertility rates of Japan). *Jinko Mondai Kenkyu (Journal of Population Problems)* 58(3): 15–44 (in Japanese).

Iwasawa, Miho, and Fusami Mita. 2007. Bansanka-to kyojikibo josei jinko-no koreika (Delayed childbearing and the changing age composition of women who desire children). *Jinko Mondai Kenkyu (Journal of Population Problems)* 63(3): 24–41 (in Japanese).

Japan Society of Obstetrics and Gynecology (JSOG) (Nihon Sanka Fujinka Gakkai). 2008. *Sanka Fujinka Yogoshu-Yogo Kaisetsushu Kaitei 2-han*. Tokyo: Kanehara-shuppan (in Japanese).

Kamata, Kenji. 2010. Chiho jichitai-ni okeru shoshikataisaku-no seisakukatei. In *Kazoku-rodoseisaku-touno Shoshikataisaku-ga Kekkon-shusshokodo-ni oyobosu Koka-ni kansuru Sogotekikenkyu: Heisei 21-nendo Sokatsu-buntan Kenkyuhokokusho (Research on policy planning and evaluation/health labour sciences research grant (H20-Seisaku-Ippan-008)*, ed. Takahashi, Shigesato, 285–311 (in Japanese).

Knudsen, L.B. 1999. Denmark-ni okeru saikin-no shussyoritsu-no doko: Shusshoritsu joshoki-no kazokuseisaku-no kage (Trans. Kamano, Saori). *Jinko Mondai Kenkyu (Journal of Population Problems)* 55(3): 3–26 (in Japanese).

Menken, Jane, and Ulla Larsen. 1986. Fertility rates and aging. In *Aging, reproduction, and the climacteric,* eds. Mastroianni, Luigi Jr. and C. Alvin Paulsen, 147–166. New York: Plenum Press.

Menken, Jane, James Trussell, and Ulla Larsen. 1986. Age and infertility. *Science* 233: 1389–1394.

Ministry of Health, Labour and Welfare (MHLW) (Koseirodosho). 2015. *Heisei 25-nen (2013) Jinko Dotai Toukei (Kakuteisu) no Gaikyo*. http://www.mhlw.go.jp/toukei/saikin/hw/jinkou/kakutei13/index.html (in Japanese).

Moriizumi, Rie. 2007. Senshin shokoku-no shussyoritsu-wo-meguru kokusaiteki doko. *Kaigai Shakaihosho Kenkyu* 160: 4–21 (in Japanese).

Moriizumi, Rie. 2010. Nihon-ni okeru shoshikataisaku-no tenkai: 1990–2010. In *Kazoku-rodoseisaku-touno Shoshikataisaku-ga Kekkon-shusshokodo-ni oyobosu Koka-ni kansuru Sogotekikenkyu: Heisei 21-nendo Sokatsu-buntan Kenkyuhokokusho (Research on policy planning and evaluation/health labour sciences research grant) (H20-Seisaku-Ippan-008)*, ed. Takahashi, Shigesato, 45–53 (in Japanese).

National Institute of Population and Social Security Research (IPSS) (Kokuritsu Shakai Hosho Jinko Mondai Kenkyujo). 2012. *Dai 14-kai Shussho Doko Kihon Chosa Dai-1 Hokokusho: Wagakuni Fufu-no Kekkon Katei-to Shusshoryoku* (*Report on the fourteenth Japanese national fertility survey in 2010: marriage process and fertility of married couples)* (Survey Series No. 29) (in Japanese).

Ohbuchi, Hiroshi, Shigesato Takahashi, Ryuichi Kaneko, Hisakazu Kato, Kohei Wada, Miho Iwasawa, and Rie Harada. 1998. Shusshoryoku hendo moderu kochiku-no tame no kiso kenkyu. *Jinko Mondai Kenkyu (Journal of Population Problems)* 54(1): 88–119 (in Japanese).

Oishi, Akiko. 2007. Funin chiryou shien-ni tsuiteno ichi kousatsu: Kazoku zokusei-no shiten-kara. In *Shoshika Kanren Shisaku-no Mitoshi-ni kansuru Kenkyu: Heisei 18-nendo Hokokusho (Research on policy planning and evaluation/health labour sciences research grant)* (H17-Seisaku-Ippan-017), ed. Takahashi, Shigesato, 86–98 (in Japanese).

Ozawa, Nobuaki, Mari Mitsui, Masashi Hanaoka, Aiko Sasaki, and Noriyoshi Watanabe. 2010. Korei shussan-to ryuzan risuku. *Sanfujinka-no Jissai (Obstetrical and Gynecological Practice)* 59(2): 167–172 (in Japanese).

Research Group for Women and the Declining Birth Rate (Shoshika-to Joseino Kenko Kenkyukai) (Nihon Iryo Seisaku Kiko). 2005. *Seisaku Teigen: Shoshika-to Josei-no Kenko (Seisaku Teigen Series, Iryoseisaku No.1)*. http://www.healthpolicy-institute.org/handout/2010-04-16_33_998301.pdf (in Japanese).

Ryder, Norman B. 1965. The cohort as a concept in the study of social change. *American Sociological Review* 30(6): 843–861.

Saito, Hidekazu, and Touko Shirakawa. 2012. *Ninkatsu Baiburu*. Tokyo: Kodansha (in Japanese).

Sato, Ryuzaburo, and Miho Iwasawa. 1998. Wagakuni-no fufu-ni okeru ninshin, shussho-no chosei: Ninshinreki-no bunseki (Reproductive intentions and fertility control behavior of Japanese married couples: Analysis of the pregnancy history). *Jinko Mondai Kenkyu (Journal of Population Problems)* 54(4): 19–45 (in Japanese).

Scheid, Teresa L., and Tony N. Brown. 2009. *A handbook of the study of mental health: social contexts, theories, and systems*, 2nd ed. Cambridge: Cambridge University Press.

Senba, Yukari. 2003. *Shoshika Taisaki-ni okeru Funin Chiryo Shien-ni tsuiteno Kenkyu (A study of support for infertility treatments and government policy toward the declining birthrate in Japan)*. Waseda University Doctoral Dissertation (in Japanese).

Senda, Yukiko. 2007. 'Birth control' to tsuma-no kekkon, shussango-no shugyokodo-no kanren. In *Shoshika Kanren Shisaku-no Koka-to Shusshoritsu-no Mitoshi-ni kansuru Kenkyu (Research on policy planning and evaluation/health labour sciences research grant) (H17-Seisaku-Ippan-017)*, ed. Takahashi, Shigesato, 71–85 (in Japanese).

Senda, Yukiko. 2011. Ninshinkito-no enki-to kodomosu: Ito sezaru kekka-to shiteno shusshoryoku teika (Increasing pregnancy attempt age and decreasing children: Fertility decline as an unintended consequence). *Jinko Mondai Kenkyu (Journal of Population Problems)* 67(4): 22–38 (in Japanese).

Senda, Yukiko. 2014. Ninshinkito-no enki-to shusshoryoku teika (Postoponent of pregnancy attempt and fertility decline). In *Nihon Jinko Gakkai Dai66-kai Taikai Hokoku Yoshi Shu:* 97–98 (in Japanese).

Shanahan, Michael J., Hofer, Scott M., and Richard A Miech. 2003. Planful competence, the life course, and the aging. In *Personal Control in Social and Life Course Contexts*, eds. Zarit, Steven H., Leonard I. Pearlin, and K. Warner Schaie, 189–211. New York: Springer.

Suzumori, Kaoru. 2004. Ninshin shoki-no Ijo. In *Hyojun Sanka Fujinkagaku*, 3rd ed, eds. Maruo, Takeshi and Takashi Okai, 317–325. Tokyo: Igaku-Shoin (in Japanese).

Takayama, Noriyuki, Hiroshi Ogawa, Hiroshi Yoshida, Fumiko Arita, Yoshihiro Kaneko, and Katsuhisa Kojima. 2000. Kekkon, ikuji-no keizai kosuto-to shusshoryoku: Shoshika-no keizaigakuteki yoin-ni kansuru ichikosatsu (The cost of marriage and child care and its effects on fertility: A note on the economic factors of below-replacement fertility in Japan). *Jinko Mondai Kenkyu (Journal of Population Problems)* 56(4): 1–18 (in Japanese).

Wood, James W. 1994. *Dynamics of human reproduction: Biology, biometry, demography*. New York: Aldine de Gruyter.

Yamaguchi, Kazuo. 2004. *Shoshika-no Kettei Yoin-to Taisaku-ni tsuite: Otto-no Yakuwari, Shokuba-no Yakuwari, Seifu-no Yakuwari, Shakai-no Yakuwari* (RIETI discussion paper series 04-J-045) (in Japanese).

Yamaguchi, Kazuo. 2009. *Waku Raifu Baransu: Jissho-to Seisaku Teigen (Work life Balance)*. Tokyo: Nihon Keizai Shinbun Shuppansha (Nikkei Publishing) (in Japanese).

Yoshimizu, Yukari. 2006. *'35-sai kara-no Shussan' wo Erabu Anatani: Jibun-de Kimeru Shussan Tekireiki*. Tokyo: Aki Shobo (in Japanese).

Chapter 3
Cohort-Specific Life Experiences Under Rapidly Changing Socioeconomic Conditions

Abstract Changes in women's family and employment behaviours and related conditions are examined for the 1960s cohort, as well as for the preceding and following cohorts. Official Japanese statistics show a declining trend in both marriage and marital fertility, as well as the indistinctness of the M-shaped curve for women's employment patterns, which both reflect the diversification of women's life course. A new lifestyle emerged among women in the 1960s cohort, which was characterised by staying single, having no children, maintaining full-time employment, and delay in social norms. Changes in education, laws, and social norms are the background for this transformation. Law/policy changes in the 1980s created workplaces that were gender equal and encouraged continuous full-time employment on their surface did not promote women's continued employment while they were raising children in reality, but it created public opinions that let women who remained unmarried and childless to continue working go. It was also during this time that social norms were being restructured to make social systems suitable to an aging society with an increasing lifespan. In the 1990s, there was also a change in social norms toward stigmatizing pregnancy at an advanced age because of the changing criteria used in medicine/health policy. These changes influenced the characteristics of life course of the 1960s cohort.

Keywords Women's family/employment behaviour · Labour law · Childcare leave · Social norm · Life course

3.1 Marriage and Childbearing Behaviour

As seen in the previous chapter, the falling fertility rate associated with marriage decline since the 1980s began with the 1960s cohort. As the social life-cycle was delayed, births by women in this cohort during their 20s significantly dropped. The decline in fertility was thus dictated by a change in the social life-cycle that dramatically reduced births by women in their 20s. The timing of childbearing was shifted to later in life. Why did this change occur? This chapter aims to uncover the reason.

Y. Senda, *Childbearing and Careers of Japanese Women Born in the 1960s*,
Population Studies of Japan, DOI 10.1007/978-4-431-55066-2_3

We have already confirmed the trend in the changing CTFR and age profile of fertility among cohorts (Fig. 2.1) in the previous chapter. Here, we will take closer look at the changes in women's life courses in that period.

Figure 3.1 shows the estimated fluctuations of the never-married rate and the estimated number of children per woman by year of birth. The figures are based on the actual statistics, up to 2010, and on the medium fertility/medium mortality projection by the National Research Institute of Population and Social Security (IPSS) for 2011 forward.

In brief, Fig. 3.1 exhibits declines in both the marriage rate and marital fertility in the 1960s cohort. Comparing those who were born in 1960 to those born in 1970, the never-married rate at age 50 increased from 9.4 to 15.3 %. The never-married rate has consistently shown an upward trend since the 1960s. Those who were born in 1960s were the first generation to experience marriage decline in Japan.

Figure 3.1 also shows the estimated number of children per woman by year of birth. We will examine the characteristics of marital and fertility behaviours for the 1960s cohort. Here, we will illustrate them by comparing the 1960 and 1970 cohorts. Women who had three or more children accounted for 25.1 % of all women born in 1960. This percentage dropped by about 9 points for those who were born in 1970. Having two children was most common among women who were born in 1960, accounting for 43.5 % of the total population. This percentage dropped by about 7 points for those who were born in 1970, although having two children was still the mode. Among those who were born in 1960, those who had one child accounted for 13.9 % of the total. This percentage rose by about 5 points

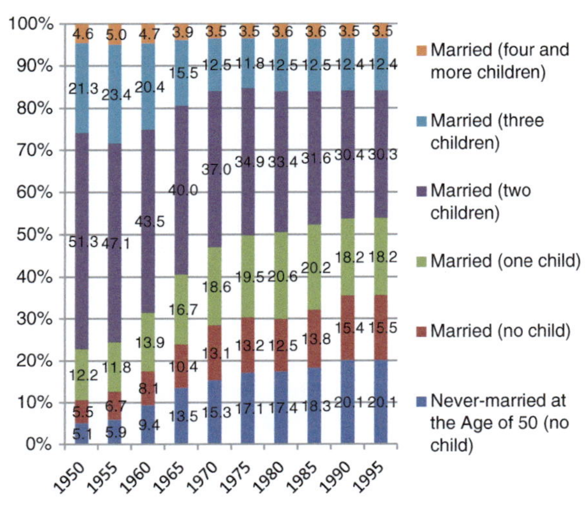

Fig. 3.1 Estimated trends in women's never-married rate at age 50 and the estimated distribution of the number of children per woman by cohort. *Source* IPSS (2012b), based on the medium fertility/medium mortality projection. 1950–1960 cohort: real statistics. 1965–1995 cohort: real statistics and the medium fertility/medium mortality projection

for those who were born in 1970. The percentage of married women who did not have children increased from 8.1 % in 1960 to 13.1 % in 1970. The percentage of never-married women increased from 9.4 % in 1960 to 15.3 % in 1970. Since it is rare for never-married women in Japan to have children, we can assume that never-married women had no children. Therefore, 17.5 % of all women who were born in 1960 had no children. This percentage increased by 10.9 points for those who were born in 1970, accounting for 28.4 % of the total.

Fertility behaviour and work behaviour affect, or are linked to, each other. In the following, we will first examine how female employment behaviour has changed with the times. We will then examine the backgrounds that brought these changes in the fertility and employment behaviours of women in Japan, focusing on the 1960s cohort.

3.2 Employment Among Women

In the late-20th century, Japan's industrial structure drastically shifted, in the course of modernization, from one centred on the primary sector to a structure centred on the secondary sector, and finally to one centred on the tertiary sector.

This economic change was accompanied by a change in the manner of women's work. Before the 1950s, women mainly worked in their family businesses in primary industries. In the 1960s, the high economic growth expanded employment opportunities for women in secondary industries. In the 1970s and later, tertiary industries further grew. Through these industrial shifts, women's labour force participation dropped once before rising: the number of women working for their families decreased in the 1960s, and then the numbers of employed women increased. Today, women exhibit a higher rate of labour force participation than immediately after the war ended in 1945.

The changes women's labour force participation by age, marital status, and employment status will now be decomposed. The number of middle-aged and married self-employed workers fell during the 1950s and 1960s. The amount of young and non-married women working as regular employees has grown since the 1970s. The number of middle-aged and married women who enter the labour market as non-regular employees, such as part-time workers, has increased since the 1970s.

Takenaka (1989) looked at the history of female labour over the period from 1945 to the 1980s. She divided the periods into three parts, based on the state of industry: Period I (1945–1960), Period II (1960–1973) and Period III (1973–1980s). Period I was the stage on which the capitalistic production style evolved from the post-war turmoil. Period II was the high-growth period, when the centre of the industrial structure shifted from primary to secondary industries. Period III was the time during which when the centre of the industrial structure moved from secondary industries to tertiary industries during the low-growth period following the 1973 oil crisis. It was also the time when legislation related to female workers significantly changed. Although Takenaka (1989) could not observe this, after her Period III, Japan experienced a bubble economy in late-1980s, as well as its burst and a long recession that continues through today. This period, between the 1990s and the present, is often referred to as the 'Lost Decades' (Aoki 2012).

Takenaka's periodization corresponds to the life stages of the 1960s cohort as follows. Period I was when their parents' generation grew up, began working, and married. Period II was their childhood. Period III was when they graduated school and became employed. For many women from the first half of the cohort, it was also a period for occupational career development and family development, such as marriage and childbirth. The late-1960s cohort experienced marriage and childbirth after the 'Lost Decades' started.

3.3 Continued Employment Among Women

Women are more likely to suspend their occupational career during the periods of marriage, childbirth, and childcare (Hakim 2000). Analyses using a variety of indicators have estimated that the percentage of women who keep their regular employment during marriage, childbirth, and childcare is around 20 %[1] (Tanaka 1996; Shintani 1998; Nagase 1999; Ohsawa and Suzuki 2000; Kawaguchi 2001). This rate of continued employment has not changed significantly over time (Tanaka 1996). However, since the mid-1990s, the timing of when women leave their jobs had shifted from their marriage to the birth of their first child (Imada 1996; Senda 2002).

Here, the official statistics for female employment continuity will be examined. From 2005 to 2009, the number of women who continued to work after having their first child was only 26.8 % (Fig. 3.2). The percentage of those who maintained their employment did not increase over these 20 years. On the other hand, the average length of service increased over those same years, from 6.8 years in 1985 to 8.9 years in 2012 (*Basic Survey on Wage Structure*). Looking at the breakdown by years of service, in 1985 the percentage of women in the workplace for 4 years or less was 53.3 %; for 5–9 years, 21.8 %; and for 10 years or more, 24.9 %. In 2012, the number of women with 4 years or less of service was 44.5 %; with 5–9 years, 23.2 %; and with 10 years or more, 32.2 % (Fig. 3.3). These statistics suggest that the rise in the average length of service seems to have been due to a decrease in the percentage of women with 4 years or less of service, and a rise in the percentage of women with 10 years or more. Since there has not been any change in the percentage of women continuing to work after giving birth, the

[1]Kanai (2010) indicated that the percentage of women who keep their regular employment through childbirth and childcare was 10 %, referring to a survey conducted by the Cabinet Office in 2006. However, this finding would not be reliable here because the survey was web-based and the sample was non-representative.

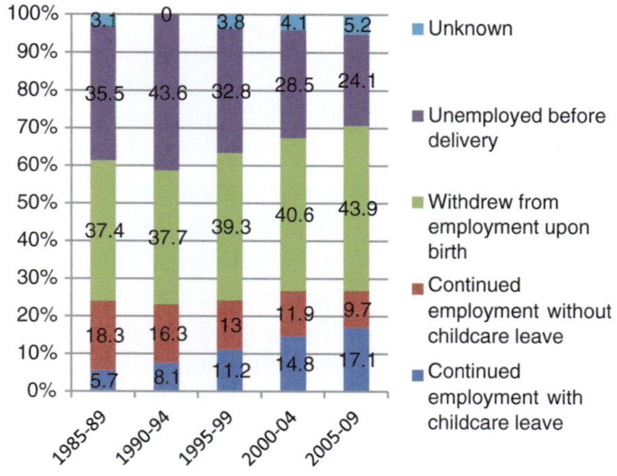

Fig. 3.2 Employment state at the timing of the first birth by the year of the first birth. *Source* IPSS (2012a)

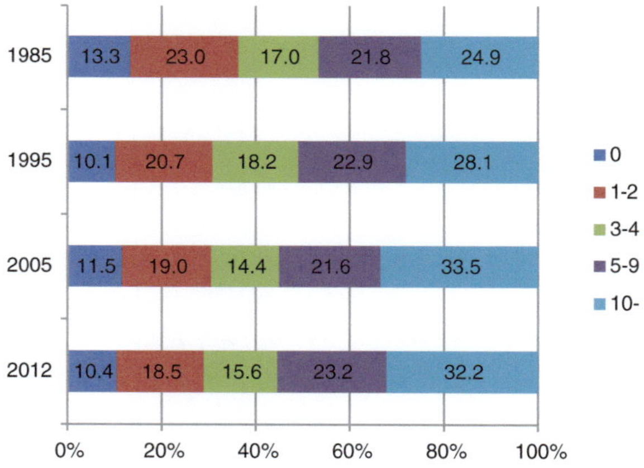

Fig. 3.3 Disribution of women's length of service. *Data Basic Survey on Wage Structure*

rise in the average length of service and the increase in people staying on the job for 10 or more years are likely due to women who never married or who married later in life. These changes appeared after the 1960s cohort began to enter the workplace.

3.4 Changes in Female Labour as Seen in the *Employment Status Survey*

In the following section, we will track historical changes in female labour by using the official data from the *Employment Status Survey*, conducted by the Statistic Bureau, Ministry of Public Management, Home Affairs, Posts and Telecommunications. For this type of attempt, the *Labour Force Survey*, which is also conducted monthly by the same office, is often used. However, since the method used in the *Labour Force Survey* changed in 1967, it is not possible to get data of detailed employment status from earlier periods. On the other hand, the *Employment Status Survey* has the advantage of allowing us to use such kind of date from 1958, although the drawback is that the survey is conducted only every three or five years.

Employment status among women by age classification is shown by year, from 1956 to 2012, in Figs. 3.4, 3.5, 3.6, 3.7, 3.8, 3.9, 3.10, 3.11, 3.12, 3.13, 3.14, 3.15, 3.16, 3.17 and 3.18. When employment status is compared across the years, the trend in employment status can be divided into five stages (1956–1959, 1962–1974 1977–1987, 1992–1997, and 2002–present). In the following, we will examine the data from the years representing each stage. We will look at how women's employment status in each stage is related to the life stages of women in the 1960s cohort, which is the subject of this book.

Employment statuses are classified in a stratified manner as follows. First, there is a distinction between 'Engaged in work' and 'Not engaged in work'. The former is divided into 'Mainly engaged in work' and 'Engaged in work on the side'.

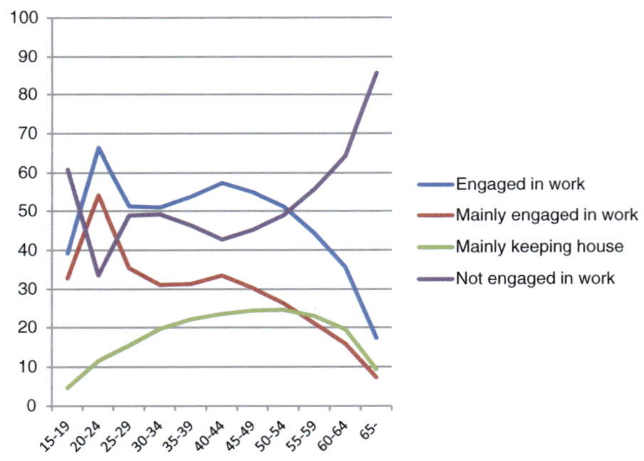

Fig. 3.4 Women's employment status by age classification: 1956

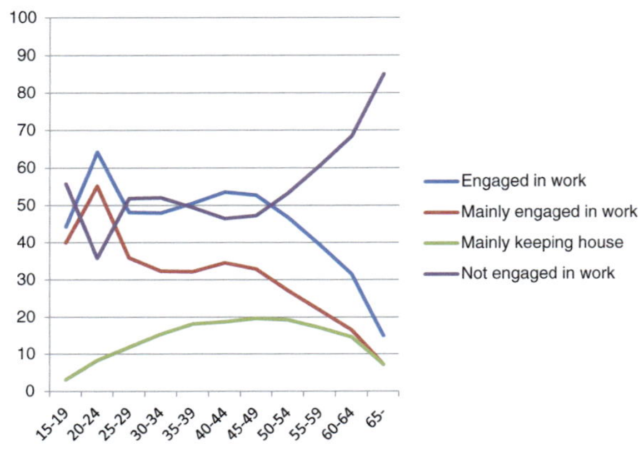

Fig. 3.5 Women's employment status by age classification: 1959

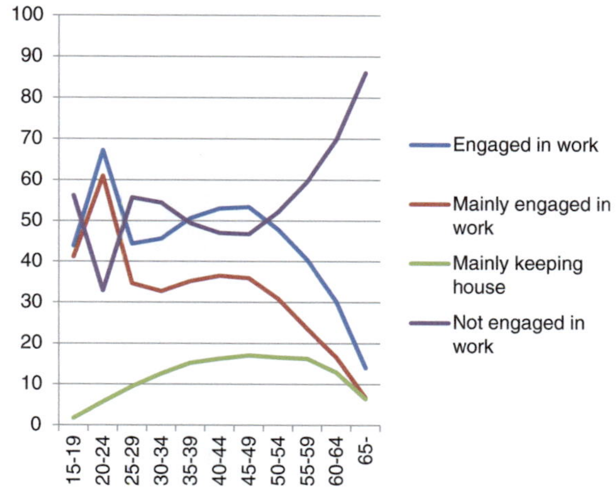

Fig. 3.6 Women's employment status by age classification: 1962

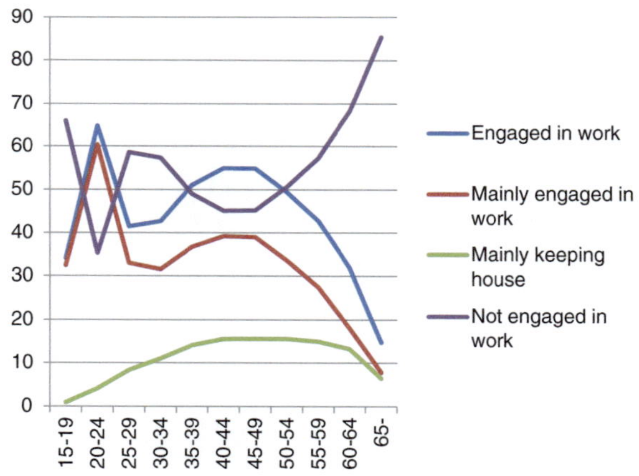

Fig. 3.7 Women's employment status by age classification: 1965

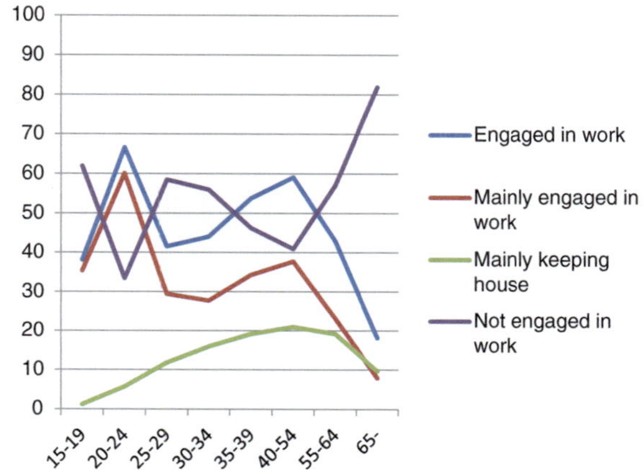

Fig. 3.8 Women's employment status by age classification: 1968

Fig. 3.9 Women's employment status by age classification: 1971

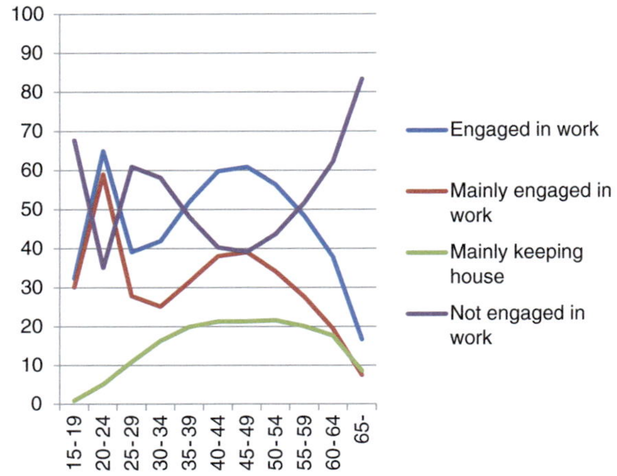

Fig. 3.10 Women's employment status by age classification: 1974

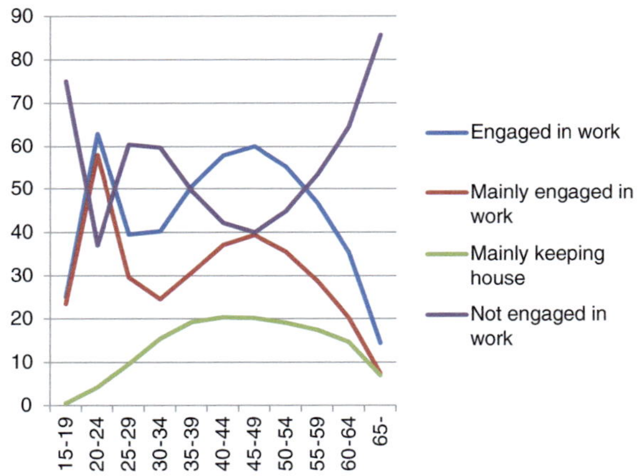

Fig. 3.11 Women's employment status by age classification: 1977

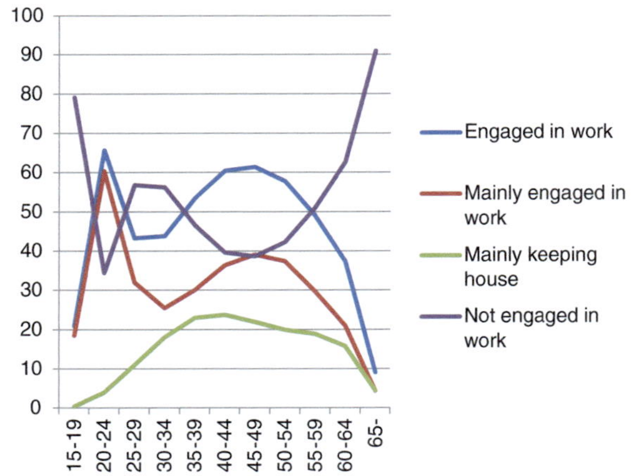

Fig. 3.12 Women's employment status by age classification: 1982

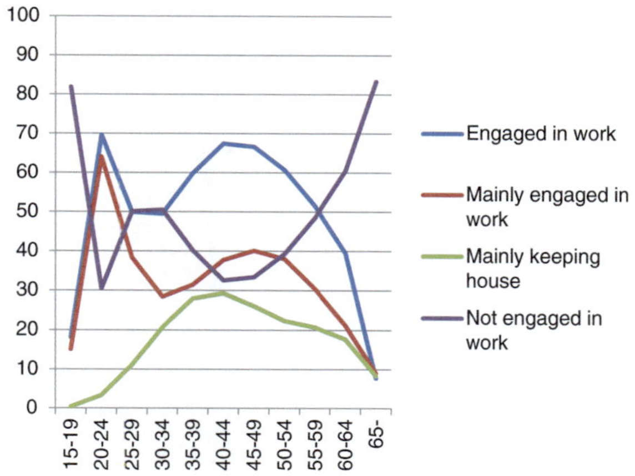

Fig. 3.13 Women's employment status by age classification: 1987

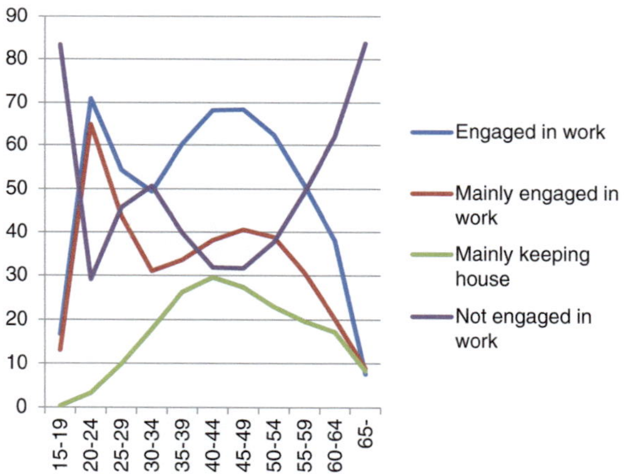

Fig. 3.14 Women's employment status by age classification: 1992

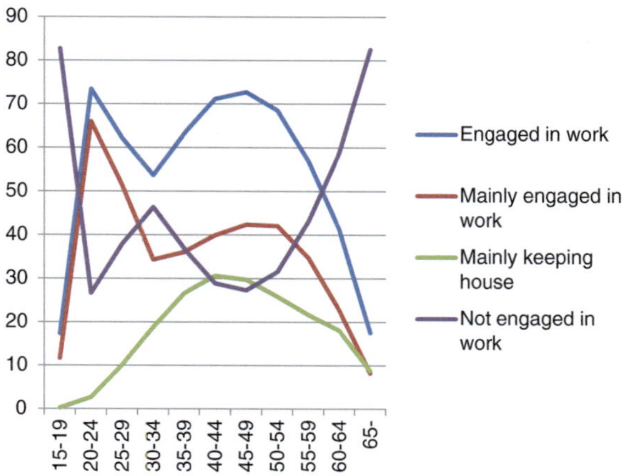

Fig. 3.15 Women's employment status by age classification: 1997

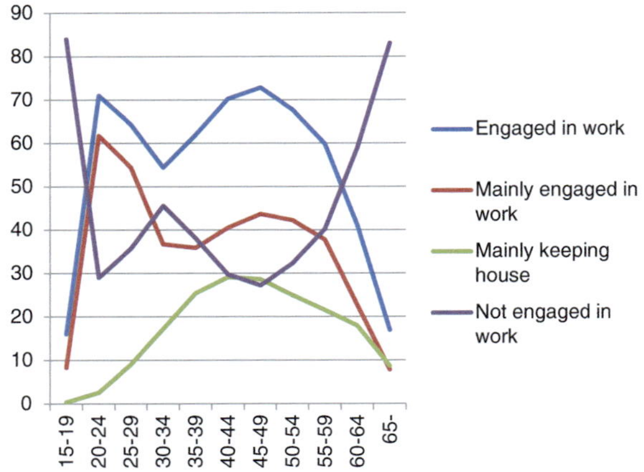

Fig. 3.16 Women's employment status by age classification: 2002

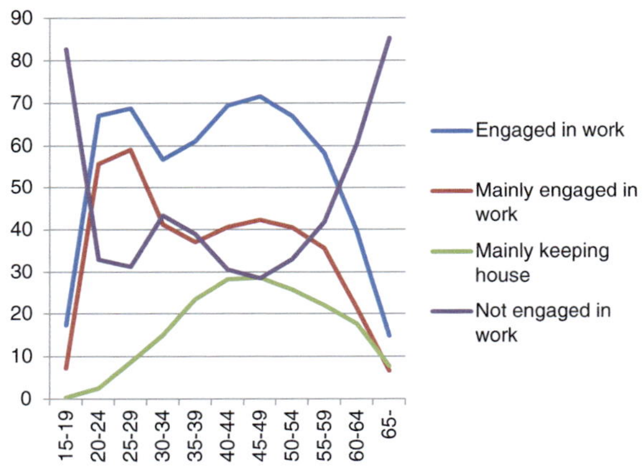

Fig. 3.17 Women's employment status by age classification: 2007

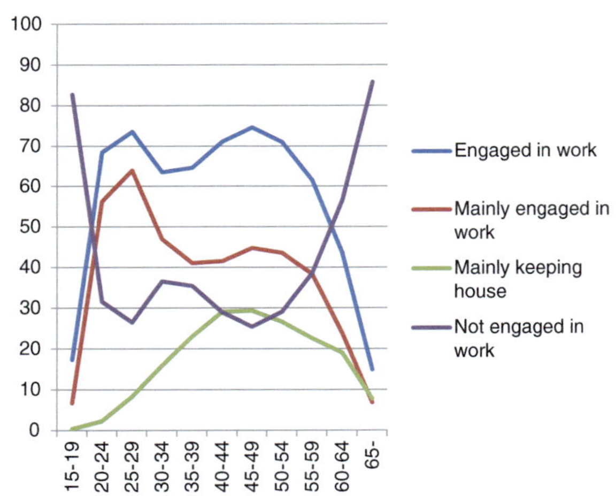

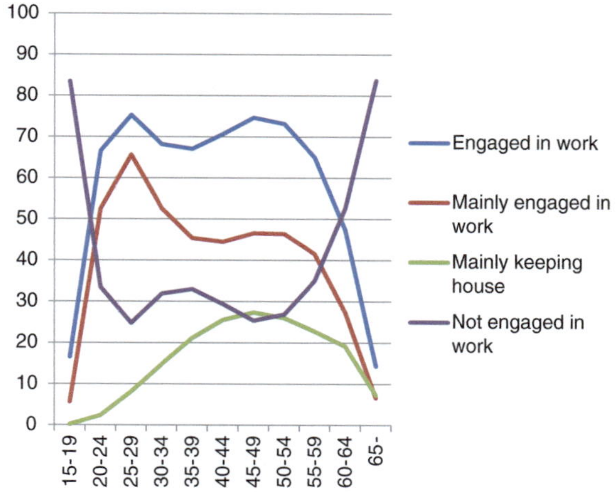

Fig. 3.18 Women's employment status by age classification: 2012

'Engaged in work on the side' is again classified into three categories: 'Mainly keeping house', 'Mainly attending school', and 'Mainly doing something else'. When looking at Figs. 3.4, 3.5, 3.6, 3.7, 3.8, 3.9, 3.10, 3.11, 3.12, 3.13, 3.14, 3.15, 3.16, 3.17 and 3.18, first focus on the two lines for 'Engaged in work' and 'Not engaged in work', in order to grasp the tendency toward workforce participation in this age profile. Next, focus on the two lines for 'Engaged in work' and 'Mainly engaged in work' or 'Mainly engaged in work' and 'Mainly keeping house', which represent women's working styles.

The first stage is represented by the period between 1956 and 1959. During this period, the employment rate was highest at 65 % for those aged 20–24. It was lowest at 50 % for those aged 25–34 (excluding those aged 15–19, who were of school age). The employment rate changed very little among those aged 25 and older. The class of people who were 'Not engaged in work' and those 'Engaged in work' competed with each other between the ages of 25 and 34. Those 'Mainly keeping house' became smaller as the women worked in their family businesses dwindled.

The second stage is represented by the period between 1962 and 1974. During the decade of the 1960s, the employment rate was at its highest, at 65 % among those aged 20–24. It was at its lowest, 40 %, among those aged 25–34. Referring to the decade of the 1950s, the difference between the highest and lowest points grew by 10 points. This probably had to do with the fact that the industrial structure was shifting from primary industries (which mainly consisted of self-employed workers) to secondary industries (mainly consisting of employed labour). Mothers of the 1960s cohort showed a stronger tendency to quit working upon marriage than seen in prior generations. The class of people who were 'Not engaged in work' was larger than the class of those 'Engaged in work' between the ages of 25 and 34. Those 'Mainly keeping house' became smaller.

In 1971 and 1974, the trend in which the employment rate was highest among those aged 20–24 and lowest among those aged 25–34 was almost the same as it had been in the 1960s, with the exception that the employment rate fell to below 40 % among those aged 25–29. This change occurred because more women left their jobs following marriage or childbirth.

The most significant new trend in this decade was that the employment rate again increased among those in their 40s. This is the emergence of the so-called 'M-shaped curve'. During this period, leaving a job once at the time of marriage and then becoming reemployed later became the standard life course for Japanese women. Mothers of the members of the 1960s cohort were the first generation to begin balancing work and childcare, by way of quitting their jobs and then regaining employment. Women in their 40s mainly worked in their spare time, possibly as part-time employees. This corresponds to the difference in rates between the 'Engaged in work' and 'Mainly engaged in work' categories, which was largest among those aged 40–49, by 20 points. Also, those 'Mainly keeping house' became larger in their 40s or later. The members of the 1960s cohort grew into adults while watching their mothers choose a new life course.

The third stage represents the period between 1977 and 1987. During this period, the valley of the M-shaped curve (the age group with the lowest employment rate) moved toward those aged 30–34. This shift was caused by the fact that fewer women were leaving their jobs at the ages of 25–29 and more women began leaving their jobs at the ages of 30–34. Moreover, among those aged 30–34, the ratio of people who were 'Mainly engaged in work' gradually became bigger. In addition, the valley became shallower as the employment rate, which had been previously 40 % during the period represented by the valley, rose to 50 %. One out of every two women was engaged in work, even in her early 30s.

This change occurred for two reasons. First, the timing at which women left their jobs began to shift from marriage to childbirth. Second, more women in the 1948–1957 cohorts (mainly the 1950s cohort) postponed marriage compared to women in the earlier cohorts as shown in Table 3.1.

This period was also the time when Japanese women developed their own occupational careers while getting the feel for the trend toward longer employment periods due to the changes in the timing among elder women for marriage and leaving the workforce. The middle segment of the 1960s cohort graduated from high school, and the majority of them began working, during this period. They may have subsequently witnessed changing behaviour patterns in work, marriage, and childbirth among the elder women at their workplace.

The fourth stage is represented by the years between 1992 and 1997. During this period, women in the 1958–1967 cohorts (mainly the 1960s cohort) were 25–34 years old. The time had finally come for the 1960s cohort to make decisions concerning marriage, childbirth, and employment. Although the age group at the valley of the M-shaped curve was still those women aged 30–34, the valley became even shallower as the employment rate during this period rose to 55 %.

Table 3.1 Trends in SMAM (the singulate mean age at marriage)

	Wife	Husband
1947	22.9	26.1
1950	23.0	25.9
1955	23.8	26.6
1960	24.4	27.2
1965	24.5	27.2
1970	24.2	26.9
1975	24.7	27.0
1980	25.2	27.8
1985	25.5	28.2
1990	25.9	28.4
1995	26.3	28.5
2000	27.0	28.8
2005	28.0	29.8
2010	28.8	30.5
2013	29.8	30.9

Data Vital Statistics

Also, the number of women who were 'Mainly engaged in work' in their late 20s and early 30s began to increase. This meant that more women in the 1960s cohort than before began to prioritise their continued employment rather than marriage and childbirth at the point in their lives when they were supposed to be of a suitable age for marriage and childbirth.

The fifth stage covers 2002 to the present (the data is up to 2012). The valley of the M-shaped curve was extended to include those aged 30–39. The valley also became increasingly shallower. Although it is still an M-shaped curve, the valley became less distinct because the gap between the two peaks and the bottom reached less than 10 points in 2012. Another characteristic of the fifth stage is that women stopped leaving their jobs at ages 25–29. These women of 1970s cohort now continued to work into their late 20s. Although they still left their jobs for childbirth, the number of women who chose to continue working during their supposedly childbearing years also increased as they found the means of continuing to work with or without a child.

As for the 1960s cohort, they were 31–40 years old in 2000 and 41–50 in 2010. The ratio of those who were 'Mainly engaged in work' continued to increase. In 2002, the lowest age group in this stage were those women aged 35–39 (1963–1967), by 37 %. This lower level was even shallower than before. In 2012, the bottom of 'Mainly engaged in work' category was those aged 40–44 (1968–1972), by 44 %, while the ratio of those women aged 45–49 (1963–1967) was 47 %. It is plausible to say that more of the women in the 1960s cohort than before continued to work even into middle age.

3.5 Popularisation of Higher Education

A woman's academic background is both a matter of her life course and an influence on the path her life course takes. Using this perspective, we will look at the academic careers of women and at gender differences in school enrolments in Japan.

The changes in the percentage of students who advanced to higher education in post-war Japan are shown, by gender, in Fig. 3.19. There was a gap in the high school enrolment rate between men and women in the late 1950s. While the rate was about 60 %, which was not so high, among men, it was less than 50 % among women. The difference in the high school enrolment rate was likely to have been even greater prior to that the 1950s. Thus, there was a gender difference in the level of educational attainment for the generation of the parents of the 1960s cohorts.

The gender differences in the high school enrolment rate disappeared in the 1960s. The enrolment rate continued to increase, and mostly stabilised at around 95 % by 1980. The 1960s cohort was a generation educated after it become common for both men and woman to advance to high school.

However, the gender difference in the four-year college enrolment rate remained. To this date, the enrolment rate among men has been consistently higher. That said, the magnitude of the gender difference in school enrolment rates varies by period. The college enrolment rate in the first half of the 1950s was about 10 %, even among men, and 3 % among women. Since the enrolment rate was also low among men, the gender difference was not as large. Since then, the enrolment rate among men continued its consistent rise until the 1970s, reaching 40 % by 1980. Although the rate increased among women during the same period, it was still 10 % in 1980. The gender difference in the college enrolment rate during this time was about 30 points, the largest difference of all periods for which data were collected. This trend continued through the 1980s.

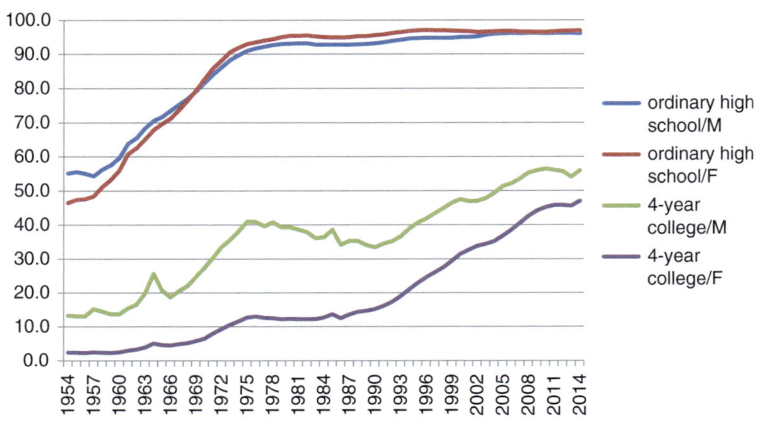

Fig. 3.19 Changes in school enrolment rates by gender. *Data School Basic Survey*

This was the period in which the 1960s cohort graduated from high school. While attending college had become quite common among men during 1980s, it was still rare for women to attend college, even though it was not as unusual as before.

Later, the college enrolment rate among women sharply increased after the 1990s, reaching almost 50 % by 2014. The rate among men was a little over 50 %. Therefore, going to college has become common among both men and women today, and the gender difference in school enrolment rate has also become quite small.

3.6 Labour Law and Women

Along with an individual's academic background, social conditions, especially social norms, also influence that individual's work behaviour. We will first look at the law, which is the formal institution of social norms.

3.6.1 Prohibition of Gender Discrimination

Japan ratified the UN Convention on the Elimination of All Forms of Discrimination against Women in 1985. As a requirement for ratifying this convention, Japan began working to eliminate discrimination against women in employment, enacting the Equal Employment Opportunity Law (EEOL) in 1986. Revising the Working Women Welfare Act (1972), the EEOL stipulated the employer's obligation to take efforts not to discriminate against women when recruiting, hiring, placing, and promoting workers, as well as efforts to implement measures for health management for expecting and nursing mothers (Rodokijunchosakai 1986).

The 1999 revision to the EEOL turned the employer's obligation to take effort not to discriminate against women into obligations with penalties. In addition, it stipulated the employer's obligation to take efforts to implement countermeasures for sexual harassment against women, and allowed the Minister of Labour to publish the names of companies that violated the prescribed prohibitions on discrimination against women (Rodokijunchosakai 1998).

The 2007 revision to the EEOL became a bilateral ban prohibiting discrimination against men as well as women. It also prohibited discrimination in matters such as demotion, changes in job descriptions, changes in employment status, retirement incentives, and labour-contract renewals. Furthermore, new provisions were established to prohibit 'indirect discrimination' as well as to prohibit disadvantageous treatment for pregnancy and childbirth. Implementing countermeasures against sexual harassment toward either sex became obligatory. The Ministry of Health, Labour and Welfare is now allowed to publish the names of companies that violated these gender discrimination prohibitions or that have neglected the sexual harassment measures or maternal health management measures. A non-penal fine is now imposed on companies that violate these regulations (Rodochosakai 2006).

3.6.2 Childcare Leave

During the 1960s, the workplaces in which female employees balanced work and family became subject to employment management. The government-owned Japan Telecommunications Workers' Union and the Nippon Telegraph and Telephone Public Corporation [NTTPC, privatised into the current Nippon Telegraph and Telephone (NTT)] began discussions in the early 1960s, and signed a collective agreement on childcare leave in 1965. 'This was the first case in which a Japanese company officially acknowledged that women will continue to work through marriage, childbirth, and childcare' (Hagiwara 2008: 179). In 1975, a law was enacted to provide childcare leave for women in specific professions, such as female teachers at compulsory education schools, nurses at medical and social welfare facilities, and nursery teachers. This law can be regarded as an official acknowledgement by the Japanese government that women will continue working through marriage, childbirth, and childcare, as long as they held a professional job such as a NTTPC telephone operator, public school teacher, or nurse in the public sector.

In contrast, it was some time later when the law realised universal childcare leave and the right of all workers to take time off from work to raise children. Although there was some consideration of legislating childcare leave in the 1980s by incorporating the EEOL, it was not successful (Akamatsu 2003). Success came in 1991 with the Childcare leave Law (CCLL). It was more of a 'shock doctrine' in response to the TFR falling all the way to 1.57 in 1989, as discussed in the previous chapter.

The CCLL guarantees a period of childcare leave as a consecutive term until the child reach one year of age, and was available once per child. The CCLL also guaranteed mothers who had not taken childcare leave the right to demand that their employer exempt overtime work exceeding 24 h per month or 150 h per year until the child reached one year of age (Ministry of Labour, Women's Bureau, Women's Welfare Division 1991).

The CCLL added provisions related to family-care leave in the 1999 revision, changing its name to the Child Care and Family Care Leave Law (CCFCLL) (Rodokijunchosakai 1998). The CCFCLL has been revised several times since then.

The 2001 revision addressed the age of children for whom parents received childcare measures from their employers, such as shorter work hours, and raised it from less than one-year old to less than three-years old. It also allowed fathers to request an exemption from overtime in excess of 24 h per month or 150 h per year from their employers. It imposed the obligation on employers to make efforts to introduce a leave system that allowed parents to care for pre-school children as well as the obligation to consider the childcare or family-care situations when transferring the worker (Rodohoreikenkyukai 2002).

In the 2005 revision, it became possible for parents to take childcare leave until the child turns one-and-a-half-years old if that child could not be admitted to a nursery school even after the request had been made. The revision also made it mandatory for employers to give parents time off (five days per year) to care for their children (Japan Personnel Management & Safety Information Center 2012).

The 2010 revisions to the law mandated that employers establish a short-time work schedule for workers with children aged three years or younger. In addition, it introduced the Papa & Mama Childcare leave Plus System, which stipulated that, when both parents take childcare leave, the period of childcare leave be extended until the child turns one year and two months old. The period was extended by two months compared to when only one of the parents took childcare leave (in which case the allowed length of childcare leave remained the same as before: until the child turned one-year old) (Rodoshinbunsha 2010).

3.6.3 Childcare Leave Benefits

Neither the CCLL nor CCFCLL mandated that the employer pay wages to workers during childcare leave. However, since workers taking leave would be stranded without pay, a system was established in 1995 to use the employment insurance system as a financial resource for paying childcare leave benefits (MHLW 2013). I will itemize the main point below:

1995: Provision of the basic allowance of childcare leave benefits (20 % of the pre-leave wage) and the return-to-work benefits (5 %).

2000 Revision: Provision of the basic allowance of childcare leave benefits (30 % of the pre-leave wage) and the return-to-work benefits (10 %).

2007 Revision: Provision of the basic allowance of childcare leave benefits (30 % of the pre-leave wage) and the return-to-work benefits (20 %).

2009 Revision: Provision of 50 % of the pre-leave wage throughout the childcare leave.

2014 Revision: 67 % of the pre-leave wage up to the 180th day, And the Provision of 50 % of the pre-leave wage from the 181st day forward.

These benefits also include an exemption from social insurance premiums.

3.6.4 Revision of the Labour Standards Act Provisions on Pregnancy

From its first legislation in 1947, the Labour Standard Law already included provisions for protecting pregnant women and maternal leave. In 1998, some revisions were made. The term for prenatal leave was extended from 10 weeks to 14 weeks in the case of a multiple pregnancy. The term for postpartum leave remained at 8 weeks (Rodokijunchosakai 1998).

3.6.5 Worker Dispatching Act

The Japanese labour system experienced another change in 1980s: the legalization of worker dispatching, which had been prohibited since 1947. The system began under tight regulations. However, these regulations have gradually been relaxed to allow worker-dispatching agencies to handle almost all types of jobs.

The Worker Dispatching Act (WDA) was enacted in 1986. The system allowed staffing agencies to execute a contract that temporarily dispatched its own employees with specific skills to a company that temporarily required such human resources. The initial WDA provided that worker dispatching is legal only for the specified 26 specialist jobs, such as information-processing system work, interpretation work, secretarial work, and filing work.

The worker dispatching system thus started as 'restricted in principle'. It then immediately shifted to 'unrestricted in principle' upon the revision of the WDA in 1992. However, whereas there was no restriction to the dispatch term for specialised work, the dispatch term for general work was limited to a maximum of three years. The 2012 revision somewhat tightened regulations by limiting the dispatch term for the 26 specialist jobs to a maximum of three years, and basically prohibited the dispatch of day labourers (Tokyo Metropolitan Labour Consultation Center 2013).

3.7 The Impact of the Development of Laws on Female Employment Behaviour

An important turning point in a woman's life course is when she must decide whether to continue working or quit after marriage and childbirth. Several of the studies on women's life courses that have been conducted since the late 1980s have centred on this topic (Economic Planning Agency 1987; National Institute of Employment and Vocational Research 1988; Japan Institute for Labour Policy and Training 2006). These studies were all questionnaire surveys that used the retrospective method.

We will examine one of these studies. The JILPT (2006) compared women's continuous employment between the 1950–1960 cohorts, who began working before the EEOL, and the 1961–1975 cohorts, who began working after the EEOL. No difference was found in the continued employment rate among the women who experienced childbirth in those two cohorts. However, there was a difference between the conditions for women who continued working. In the 1950–1960 cohorts, the continuous employment rate was higher among professional women, defined as those in medical, education, or social welfare occupations as well as those in the public sector. Within the 1961–1975 cohorts, more women continued to work under a broader range of occupations. These changes would be due to the popularisation of the childcare leave system among private companies. Meanwhile, the continuous employment rate declined for those who worked as professional workers, who had exhibited a higher continuous employment rate in the past.

In the 1990s, researchers began studying women's life courses by conducting panel surveys. The first panel survey in Japan, the *Japanese Panel Survey of Consumers* (JPSC), was initiated by the Institute for Research on Household Economics. It began in 1993 by initially targeting women aged 24–34 (i.e., born between 1959 and 1969). The survey is conducted every year, and aims to shed light on women's living conditions based on household finances, work behaviour, and family relationships. By including additional cohorts, the survey aids the understanding of the life courses of the younger generations born after 1970. Since then, panel surveys have been implemented elsewhere as well. Many of them are conducted by the Ministry of Health, Labour and Welfare.[2]

In the following paragraphs, the findings from these studies will be summarised. Laws such as the EEOL and CCLL, established between the late 1980s and the early 1990s, were supposed to create women-friendly work environments and promote their continued employment. The effects of the laws are accordingly one of the focuses of the panel studies. However, the results of the panel studies revealed that the percentage of women who continued to work after childbirth did not increase, even in those cohorts that should have benefited from these laws.

Abe (2005) analysed the JPSC and concluded that CCLL's effect was very limited. That is, childcare leave takers were limited to women who would continue their employment even if no childcare leave system was available. Therefore, Abe concluded that CCLC did not expand the potential of continuous employment for women.

Nishimura (2014) also analysed the JPSC. She summarised her findings to state that there was no evidence to confirm the trend that more women were continuing to work after childbirth compared to the prior generation, even among those who were born in the 1970s.

---

[2]These following panel surveys were conducted by MHLW: *The Longitudinal Survey of Newborns in the 21st Century* surveys children who were born in 2001 to study their lives and their parents' employment status. In 2010, they added a group of children born in 2010 to the panel (http://www.mhlw.go.jp/english/database/db-hw/vs03.html); *The Longitudinal Survey of Adults in the 21st Century* is a survey that aims to understand changes in matters such as marriage, childbirth, and employment among people between 20–34 years old in 2002 (born between 1968 and 1980). They added a new group of subjects, aged 20–29, in 2012 (born between 1983 and 1992) (http://www.mhlw.go.jp/english/database/db-hss/dl/shw-10.pdf).

These studies imply that efforts that only attempted to improve the work environment through law and policy would not encourage women to continue working. There were other factors that held women back from continuing to work following childbirth. In the following section, we will examine the factors that could potentially suppress women's attempts to continue working.

3.8 The Norm that 'the Mother Should Raise Children'

As described above, legal changes that aim to promote women in the workplace had barely any effect. We can assume the existence of some factor that offsets the effect of these laws. An informal institution of social norms would be a crucial factor.

In the 1960s, the Japanese government expressed the belief that mothers have the primary responsibility of bringing up their children, and that it is for the welfare of the children that their mothers raise them. The government distorted psychological hypothesis of maternal deprivation, proposed by John Bowlby, in order to create a 'scientific' ideology of motherhood stating that the healthy development of infants was founded on the formation of a stable one-to-one attachment between the mother and child (Ohinata 1988; Hagiwara 2008). Economic Planning Agency, Economic Council (1963: 132–133) also stated that 'the majority of women have the primary responsibility of childcare as a mother, and that children, especially those under the age of three, should be individually cared for by loving relatives'. These statements were the origin of the so-called 'myth of the first three years', a belief in mother's responsibility that is widespread in Japanese society even today (Makino 2004).

In line with this official ideology, women were expected to leave their jobs upon childbirth. The government tried to reduce the number of nursery users by tightening the admission criteria (Hagiwara 2008), because there was no use in encouraging women to work over the long term. Part-time, non-regular work systems were instituted to utilize the labour of women re-entering the workspace after their childcare period.

At the same time, the mass media depicted the ideal image of home and the mother-child relationship, and the public accepted it (Sakamoto 1997). As television became a common household feature, the NHK, the public broadcaster in Japan, began broadcasting the educational entertainment program '*Okaasan to Issho*' (with mother) in 1959. The title sums up the message that 'children should be with their mother' and 'children should be brought up by their mothers'.

These social conditions provided the environment in which the members of the 1960s cohorts grew up. They were the first generation that was mainly raised by their mothers. It was during this era that a new norm permeated Japanese society.

3.9 Weakened Age Norms

3.9.1 The Gradual Disappearance of Suitable Age for Marriage

Aging and longevity are two additional aspects of social change that accompany modernization. As mortality decreases and the expected lifespan expands, there has been pressure to restructure social systems to cope with an aging society. For example, The Economic Planning Agency (1986) announced the arrival of the 'era of the 80-year life' in the mid-1980s. It laid out the challenges and directions for building economic systems, such as employment and social security systems, by adjusting systems that had previously been created on the basis of a 50-year life.

The expanding lifespans of women also affects their life plans. For women in the era of the 80-year life, the agency deemed it necessary to establish a post-childcare reemployment system to create a scheme in which women retire upon marriage and childbirth and then are re-employed later in life. This is one of the sources of change in social conditions that women face.

In 1986, women in the first part of the 1960s cohort were approaching their mid-20s. They were in a pressing situation in terms of being forced to make the decision of whether or not to marry, because it was thought at the time that the suitable age for a woman to marry was up her mid-20s. Once a woman passed her mid-20s, she was deemed to have missed the time for marriage; the situation was described using the metaphor of a Christmas cake, an item that loses its value after the 25th of December (Brinton 1992). However, that was the standard for women in the era of the 50-year life. If a woman's lifespan increases due to extended life expectancy, it should also be acceptable to extend the time before marriage.

Concurrently, the enactment of the EEOL was a major part of the news at that time, and women in the early part of the 1960s cohort had just started careers that held out for gender equality. They received the prominent message of that era, which stated that the time allotted for life was longer than they had thought, and that they did not have to become housewives just because they were women.

3.9.2 Postponing Childbirth

There were also changes in the medical system related to pregnancy and childbirth in the early-1990s. The Japan Society of Obstetrics and Gynaecology currently defines one's first pregnancy at the age of 35 or older as late childbearing ('elderly primipara' in technical terminology). The criterion for late childbearing had been at 30 years old in the past, the criterion was raised to 35 years old in 1992.

Because late childbearing felt like a kind of stigma, women often believed that they should avoid it. This stigmatization emerged from the 'mother-and-baby note-book' system. The notebook is distributed, officially, among pregnant women for their medical and welfare records. Expectant mothers must bring their notebook for prenatal care and infant health examination so that they can record their results in it. Late childbearing, determined using the above-mentioned age criterion, is referred to as *marukou* in broken Japanese, because a circled (*maru*) and the Chinese character 'high' (*kou*) is stamped onto the 'mother-and-baby notebook'. The stamp ensures the notebook holder stands out when receiving health examinations and care, and broadcasts that she is out of the standard life schedule.

A childbirth in one's early 30s used to be considered 'outside the standard' before 1992. However, it became 'within the standard' after 1992, since the age criterion for late childbirth was raised from 30 to 35. It thus extended the socially acceptable timing of pregnancy by five years.

By 1992, the women of the 1960s cohort were reaching the period of childbirth. The older segment of this cohort was already facing the social deadline for childbirth. The younger segment was about at the time to begin thinking about childbirth. The aforementioned change in the age criterion meant a sudden, five-year delay in the social deadline.

Arai (2006) called this trend an 'inferior mirage phenomenon'. That is, the raised age criterion for late childbearing provide a perfect excuse for women in their late-20s to continue working or postponing marriage and childbirth (Arai 2006: 352–353).

3.10 Accepting a New Life Course

As shown in this chapter, the women of the 1960s cohort, who are the main target of this study, experienced changes in various aspects of their lives. The childhood in which they were raised was the era of the old, strict norms for suitable ages for marriage and childbirth. However, despite growing up under such norms, these women postponed both marriage and childbirth in response to changes in their social situations when they reached those ages. The 1960s cohort followed a life course in accordance with the new social life-cycle.

This means that they have lived their lives feeling anxiety and hesitation regarding the gap between the old norms and their own life courses, which were oriented toward the new norms. The fact that the books written by those women about such anxiety and hesitation have become bestsellers has been a notable phenomenon in Japanese society in recent years. Let me conclude this chapter by introducing some of representative works of such writers.

At the time at which the 1960s cohort was at their 'suitable' age for marriage, *Kekkon Shinaikamoshirenai Shokogun (I-might-not-get-married Syndrome)* (Tanimura 1990) was published. This book portrayed how many single women in the same age group had sentiments suggesting that they would stay single, and wavered wondering how single life would be. The author, who was born in 1962, was single without a child at the time.

'Makeinu' no Toboe (Howl of Losers) (Sakai 2003) was published around the time that the 1960s cohort passed their 'suitable' age for childbirth. This book deemed women who were single with no children as losers, regardless of how socially successful they were. The book indicated that the trick by which the 'losers' survived was to bow down, from the beginning, to the 'winners', who are married with children, and say 'you are superior to us'. The author was a single, childless woman born in 1966.

Soon after that book, *Su-chan* (Masuda 2006) was published. The main character, Su-chan, was a single, childless woman in her late 30s. The book positively portrayed the dispassionate everyday life of Su-chan. The author was a single, childless woman born in 1969.

Here, the message of these books will be compared with each other in the order of their publication. Tanimura (1990) depicted the anxiety and hesitation of a way of life that deviates from the norm. Sakai (2003) depicted a 'so-what' attitude toward a way of life that deviates from the old norm. Masuda (2006) depicted acceptance and an 'I'm okay with the way I am' attitude toward a way of life that deviates from the old norm. Those who followed a life course in accordance with the new social life-cycle used to feel anxiety when deviating from the old norm. However, the discourse that 'it is okay to lead such a way of life', popularised by authors who spent their 20s and 30s being tormented by this anxiety, changed the meaning of the new life course, presenting it as something that could be positively accepted.

References

Abe, Masahiro. 2005. Dare-ga ikujikyugyo-wo shutokusurunoka. In *Kosodate Setai-no Shakaihosho*, ed. National Institute of Population and Social Security Research, 243–264. Tokyo: University of Tokyo Press (in Japanese).

Akamatsu, Ryoko. 2003. *Kintoho-wo Tsukuru*. Tokyo: Keiso Shobo (in Japanese).

Aoki, Reiko. 2012. A demographic perspective on Japan's "Lost Decades". *Population and Development Review* 38: 103–112.

Arai, Yoko. 2006. *40dai Uizan-wo Hajimeta Joseitachi*. Tokyo: Joho Center Publishing (in Japanese).

Brinton, Mary. C. 1992. Christmas cakes and wedding cakes: The social organization of Japanese women's life course. In *Japanese Social Organization*, ed. Sugiyama Lebra, Takie, 79–107. Honolulu: University of Hawaii Press.

Economic Planning Agency, Economic Council (Keizaikikakucho Keizaishingikai). 1963. *Keizai Hatten-ni okeru Jinteki Noryoku Kaihatsu-no Kadai-to Taisaku*. Tokyo: Printing Bureau, Ministry of Finance (in Japanese).

Economic Planning Agency, Social Policy Bureau (Keizaikikakucho Kokuminseikatsukyoku). 1986. *Choju Shakai-no Kozu: Jinsei 80-nen Jidai-no Keizai Shakai Shisutemu Kochiku-no Hoko*. Tokyo: Printing Bureau, Ministry of Finance (in Japanese).

Economic Planning Agency, Social Policy Bureau (Keizaikikakucho Kokuminseikatsukyoku). 1987. *Atarasii Jyoseino Ikikata-wo Motomete: Choju Shakai-ni okeru Jyosei-no Raifu* Kosu. Tokyo: Printing Bureau, Ministry of Finance (in Japanese).

Hagiwara, Kumiko. 2008. *'Ikujikyushoku' Kyoyaku-no Seiritsu: Kodo Seichoki-to Kazokuteki Sekinin*. Tokyo: Keiso-Shobo (in Japanese).

Hakim, Chatherine. 2000. *Work-Lifestyle Choices in the 21st Century: Preference Theory*. New York: Oxford University Press.

Imada, Sachiko. 1996. Joshi rodo-to shugyo keizoku. *Nihon Rodo Kenkyu Zassi (The Monthly Journal of the Japan Institute of Labour)* 433: 37–48 (in Japanese).

Japan Institute for Labour Policy and Training (JILPT) (Nihon Rodo Seisaku Kenkyu Kenshu Kiko). 2006. *Shigoto-to Katei-no Ryoritsu: Ikuji-Kaigo-wo Chushinni* (Rodo Seisaku Kenkyu Hokokusho No. 64) (in Japanese).

Japan Personnel Management & Safety Information Center (Rodoanzenjohosenta). 2012. *Ikujikaigokyugyoseido-no Hayawakari* (in Japanese). http://labor.tank.jp/kaigo.html.

Kanai, Atsuko. 2010. Hataraku josei-no kyaria-toranjishion (Career transition among working women). *Nihon Rodo Kenkyu Zassi (The Monthly Journal of the Japan Institute of Labour)* 603: 44–53 (in Japanese).

Kawaguchi, Akira. 2001. Jyosei-no marijji puremiamu: Kekkon-shussan-ga shugyo-chingin-ni ataeru eikyo. *Kikan Kakei Keizai Kenkyu* 51: 63–71 (in Japanese).

Makino, Katsuko. 2004. Kodomo-no shakaika-ni miru jenda. In *Shoshika Shakai-no Kazoku-to Fukushi*, ed. Sodei Takako, 136–146. Kyoto: Minerva Shobo (in Japanese).

Masuda, Miri. 2006. *Su-chan*. Tokyo: Gentosha (in Japanese).

Ministry of Health, Labour and Welfare (MHLW) (Koseirodosho). 2013. *Ikuji Kyugyo Kyufu* (in Japanese). http://www.mhlw.go.jp/stf/shingi/2r98520000035rib-att/2r98520000035rlf_1.pdf.

Ministry of Labour, Women's Bureau, Women's Welfare Division (Rodosho Fujin-kyokyu Fujin'fukushi-ka). 1991. *Wakariyasui Ikuji Kyugyohou*. Tokyo: Yuhikaku (in Japanese).

Nagase, Nobuko. 1999. Shoshika-no yoin: Shugyokankyo-ka kachikan-no henka-ka: Kikonsha-no shugyokeitaisentaku-to shussanjiki-no sentaku (Work and childbearing choice of married women in Japan: the effects of labor practices). *Jinko Mondai Kenkyu (Journal of Population Problems)* 55(2): 1–18 (in Japanese).

National Institute of Employment and Vocational Research (NIEVR) (Koyo Shokugyo Sogo Kenkyujo). 1988. *Josei-no Shokugyo Keireki* (Shokken Chosa Kenkyu Hokokusho 77) (in Japanese).

National Institute of Population and Social Security Research (IPSS) (Kokuritsu Shakai Hosho Jinko Mondai Kenkyujo). 2012a. *Dai 14-kai Shussho Doko Kihon Chosa Dai-1 Hokokusho: Wagakuni Fufu-no Kekkon Katei-to Shusshoryoku (Report on the Fourteenth Japanese National Fertility Survey in 2010: Marriage Process and Fertility of Married Couples)* (Survey Series No. 29) (in Japanese).

National Institute of Population and Social Security Research (IPSS) (Kokuritsu Shakai Hosho Jinko Mondai Kenkyujo). 2012b. *Nihon-no Shorai Suikei Jinko: Heisei 24-nen 1-gatsu Suikei) (Population Projections for Japan: 2011–2060)* (Research Series No. 326) (in Japanese).

Nishimura, Junko. 2014. *Kosodate-to Shigoto-no Shakaigaku: Jyoseino Hatarakikata-wa Kawattaka*. Tokyo: Koubundou (in Japanese).

Ohinata, Masami. 1988. *Bosei-no Kenkyu: Sono-keisei-to Hen'you-no Katei: Dentouteki Boseikan-heno Hansho*. Tokyo: Kawashimashoten (in Japanese).

Ohsawa, Machiko, and Haruko Suzuki. 2000. Josei-no kekkon-shussan oyobi jintekishihon-no keisei-ni kansuru paneru deta bunseki: Shussan taishoku-wa wakai sedai-de hontou-ni fuete irunoka. *Kikan Kakei Keizai Kenkyu* 48: 45–53 (in Japanese).

Rodochosakai. 2006. *Kaisei Danjo Koyou Kikai Kintouhou*. Tokyo: Rodochosakai (in Japanese).

Rodohoreikenkyukai. 2002. *Ikuji Kaigo Kyugyohou Benran (Shintei)*. Tokyo: Rodohorei (in Japanese).

Rodokijunchosakai. 1986. *Danjo Koyou Kikai Kintouhou-to Kaisei Roudou Kijunhou: Hou, Kisoku, Shishin, Shikou Tsutatsu-no Taishou Kaisetsu Ketteiban*. Tokyo: Rodo Kijun Chosakai (in Japanese).

Rodokijunchosakai. 1998. *Kaisei Danjo Koyou Kikai Kintouhou, Roudou, Kijunhou, Ikuji Kaigo Kyugyohou: Ketteiban*. Tokyo: Rodo Kijun Chosakai (in Japanese).

Rodoshinbunsha. 2010. *Wakariyasui Ikuji Kaigo Kyugyohou*. Tokyo: Rodoshinbunsha (in Japanese).

Sakai, Junko. 2003. *'Makeinu' no Toboe*. Tokyo: Kodansha (in Japanese).
Sakamoto, Kazue. 1997. *'Kazoku' Imeji-no Tanjo: Nihon Eiga-ni Miru Homu Dorama-no Keisei*. Tokyo: Shinyosha (in Japanese).
Senda, Yukiko. 2002. Kikon josei-no shugyo keizoku-to ikuji shigen-no kankei: Shokushu-to shussho kohoto-wo tegakarinishite (Influence of childcare resources on the employment continuity of married women: Focusing on occupation and birth cohort). *Jinko Mondai Kenkyu (Journal of Population Problems)* 58(2): 2–21 (in Japanese).
Shintani, Yuriko. 1998. Kekkon, shussanki-no josei-no shugyo-to sono-kiteiyoin: 1980-nendai iko-no shusshokodo-no henka-tono kanren-yori (Working of women in the marriage/childbearing periods and its defined factors in relation to changes in birth behaviors from the 1980 onward). *Jinko Mondai Kenkyu (Journal of Population Problems)* 54(4): 46–62 (in Japanese).
Takenaka, Emiko. 1989. *Sengo Joshi Roudoushiron*. Tokyo: Yuhikaku (in Japanese).
Tanaka, Sigeto. 1996. Sengo Nihon-ni okeru seibetsu bungyo-no dotai: josei-no shokuba shinshutsu-to niju-no shoheki (The Changing Sexual Division of Labor in Postwar Japan: The Double Barrier against Employment of Women). *Kazoku Shakaigaku Kenkyu (Japanese Journal of Family Sociology)* 8: 151–161 (in Japanese).
Tanimura, Shiho. 1990. *Kekkon Shinai kamo Shirenai Shokogun (I-might-not-get-married Syndrome)*. Tokyo: Shufuno-tomosha (in Japanese).
Tokyo Metropolitan Labour Consultation Center (Tokyo-to Rodo Sodan Joho Senta). 2013. *Hakensaki, Hakenmoto, Hakenrodosha. Sanmi Ittai no Rodosha Haken Koza* (in Japanese). http://manabu.metro.tokyo.jp/haken/index.html.

Chapter 4
Women's Career Development Under Japanese Human Resource Management System

Abstract In the mid-1980s Japan, when those born in the 1960s started their occupational career, the Equal Employment Opportunity Law was enforced in order to prohibit gender discrimination. Corresponding to EEOL, many large companies introduced a new course-based management system for managing their white-collar employees in a superficially gender-neutral manner, typically comprising of two courses: *ippan-shoku* and *sogo-shoku.* Under this system, almost all of the women were in the *ippan-shoku* course. Their experiences would represent those of the majority of women born in the 1960s, covering a wide range of white-collar work available to young women. The author conducted two qualitative (interview) surveys and one quantitative (questionnaire) survey of white-collar workers who mainly comprised the 1960s cohort. In the one interview survey, 41 interviews were conducted and in the ohter interview survey included 50 participants. Results describe the early- and mid- careers of *ippan-shoku* women and the difference between *sogo-shoku* women and men. Although short-term service was expected, a not-negligible number of women served for a number of years. Such long-serving *ippan-shoku* employees often have the capacity to improvise tasks that were not their own, which is indispensable for smooth accomplishment of the work in the workplace. They developed such a kind of skill through their long career, with the absence of any job rotation, in their given workplace. Companies gave *ippan-shoku* workers some career development drivers, as long as they were single.

Keywords Japanese human resource management · Career development · Course-based management · Quantitative survey · Qualitative survey

4.1 Employment Behaviour of the 1960s Cohort

Around the 1980s, when women born in the 1960s cohort turned 20, changes in the way that women worked were socially important subjects. The EEOL and CCLL made people take interest in the life course in which women continued working after marriage and childbirth. Work-life balance became a popular social

Y. Senda, *Childbearing and Careers of Japanese Women Born in the 1960s*, Population Studies of Japan, DOI 10.1007/978-4-431-55066-2_4

topic. Women in the 1950s and earlier cohorts would have left their jobs upon marriage as a matter of course. For the later cohorts, however, leaving one's job upon marriage was no longer a matter of course. Whether to marry, whether to continue working when they married, whether to bear children, and whether to continue working when they bore children all became matters of an individual's choice. The women in these cohorts now had to make decisions at their own risk.

As a result, the ratio of women who chose to work instead of having children increased. Why would women choose not to have children while they continued working? Why did the ratio of women who continued working while raising children not increase, even after systems, such as the EEOL and CCLL, were introduced to support a way of work in which women could remain employed while having children? What kind of occupational career did they have? This chapter aims to answer these questions.

Briefly, Figs. 3.4–3.18 will be re-examined by focusing on the 1960s cohort. The women in the 1960s cohort grew into adults in an era in which leaving one's job at the time of marriage and then becoming re-employed later had become a woman's life course. The centre of industry had shifted from the primary sector (in which people were mainly self-employed) to the secondary and tertiary sectors (in which people were mainly employed as labour) during the previous generation, in which the number of mothers who worked as family workers and raised children decreased and the number of women who became full-time housewives after marriage and childcare increased.

It was in the early 1990s that the 1960s cohort began making choices regarding marriage, childbirth, and employment. There were two characteristics to women's employment behaviour during this time. First, more women continued to work after marriage, but left their jobs upon childbirth. Second, more women began prioritising continued employment over marriage and childbirth. As a result, they had to choose between two opposing behaviours: to quit their jobs upon childbirth, or to continue working without children. These were the choices confronting women in the 1960s cohort.

What kind of labour force did women in the 1960s cohort compose? To understand this, I need to go back in history to understand the employment management system used by Japanese companies and how women were positioned in this system.

4.2 Japanese Human Resource Management System During the Era of High Economic Growth

Large companies in Japan established the Japanese human resource management system during the era of high economic growth. It consisted of three elements: lifetime employment, seniority-based wages, and company-based trade unions (Nomura 2007).

Under the Japanese human resource management system, lifetime employment and seniority-based wages applied only to male employees, while female employees were excluded from these benefits (Yashiro 1995). Companies provided male employees with a uniform promotion up to the section chief level. Since the organizational structure of these companies was a pyramid, some employees had to be left out, and companies selected women. Human resources were managed so that women left their jobs while they were still young and before getting to the managerial level.

Under this human resource management system, men were uniformly promoted up to the section chief level, although the speed of their promotions varied based on their performance (Imada and Hirata 1995). Male workers, therefore, accepted long working hours and relocation when required by the company, and strived to win the competition for quicker promotions. Additionally, since whether an employee could be further promoted after reaching the section chief level was determined by rigorous screening, men were motivated to work as hard as required by the company in order to demonstrate a higher level of performance than their colleagues, even after being promoted to section chief. Figure 4.1 shows this promotion management model as a diagram.

Companies guaranteed male employees lifetime employment and seniority-based wages. By guaranteeing uniform promotion up to the section chief level, they made male employees compete for the fastest promotions. In order to win the competition, men dedicated themselves to work. They were supported by the family wage, guaranteed by the company, and by their spouses, who were full-time housewives.

Companies offered male workers wages that were high enough to provide for their families. If a worker had a wife and children, the company provided him an allowance to support his family (Kimoto 2004). ‘Family wage’ was one such a wage mechanism. Since companies only guaranteed men, but not women, lifetime employment and family wages, the husband, rather than the wife, became the family’s breadwinner. This is the so-called ‘male-breadwinner model’ (Kimoto 2004; Saito 2013).

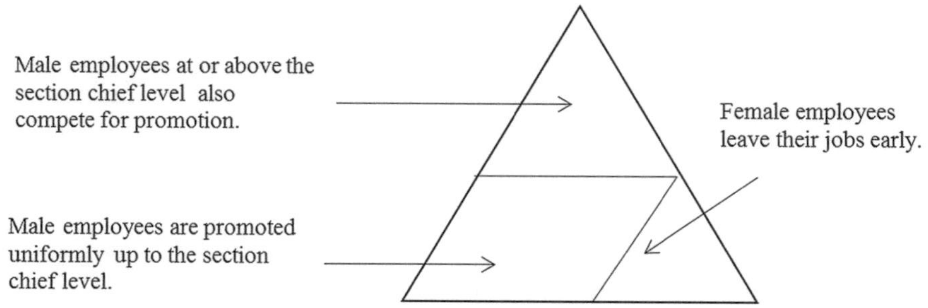

Fig. 4.1 Japanese human resource management. *Note* This figure was made in reference to Fig. 2 in Yashiro (1995: 86)

In order to earn wages to feed his family and win the promotion race, a man had to devote most of his life to work. It was his wife who supported him. Once married, the wife quit working in order to become a full-time housewife, and cared for her husband and raised children by herself. Such a gender-based division of labour was the way in which families adapted to the human resource management system of Japanese companies (Osawa 1993; Kimoto 2004; Tachibanaki 2010).

Women worked even under such employment practices. The common approach to working among women in those days was to find a white-collar/clerical job after graduating from school and to work for two to three years until they married (Tachibanaki 2010). They would perform simple tasks, such as preparing documents and making copies. Through assisting men, they learned how hard men worked at the company. After marriage, this experience became their motivation for devoting themselves to supporting their husbands, who threw themselves into work without regard for their family.

4.3 The EEOL and the Course-Based Management System

After the EEOL became effective in 1986, human resource management that was based on gender was no longer permitted. Therefore, in order to take advantage of a legal loophole, the course-based management system (*Kosu-betsu Koyo Kanri Seido*) was introduced, mainly in large companies (Watanabe 1995).[1]

Under this system, multiple career courses were established based on the difficulty of the duties the employee might be responsible for, as well as on the possibility of relocation. They typically set two courses: *sogo-shoku* (candidate for an executive position), in which the employee was in charge of planning and non-routine tasks and faced the possibility of relocating both inside and outside of Japan, and *ippan-shoku* (general clerical position), in which the employee is responsible for routine tasks without the possibility of job transfers that would require relocation. Human resource management practices—such as placement, promotion, and job training—differed depending on the employment course. In addition, the salary for *ippan-shoku* was lower than the salary for *sogo-shoku*.

In fact, most (usually all) of the *ippan-shoku* workers were women while most of the *sogo-shoku* workers were men (Koseirodosho Koji-hatsu No. 0122001, dated 22 January 2007). Thus, this system was actually intended to maintain the gendered human resource management that was practiced in the previous period.

[1]It is a historical fact that Japanese companies introduced the course-based management system at the same time that the enforcement of EEOL began (Komagawa 2014: 51). However, we should maintain some reservation about the causality between the EEOL and the course-based management system. Watanabe (1995) and Komagawa (2013) proposed that some companies had already tried to introduce merit system and sophisticated versions of the existing gender-based management system. The course-based management system might have spontaneously evolved from such efforts, rather than being created in response to the EEOL.

Table 4.1 Breakdown of women in each course and category (%)

Category of human resource management	Percentage of the course-base management system introduction	Course	Ratio occupied by women in each course	Distribution of women
Under course-based management	24.6	*Sogo-shoku*	2.5	6.1
		Semi-*sogo-shoku*	50.1	4.9
		Senmon-shoku	16.0	1.6
		Ippan-shoku	74.6	81.3
		Other	18.8	6.1
Sub total				100.0
Not under course-based management	75.4			
Total	100.0			

Source Japan Institution of Workers' Evolution (1994)

However, since it was not based on gender in theory, it was justified on the basis that *sogo-shoku* employees were responsible for more advanced tasks or had greater experience due to job transfers and relocation.

That said, in terms of their number, companies that introduced the course-based management system were a minority. Only 24.6 % of companies [2]introduced the course-based management system (Table 4.1). However, the course-based management system was regarded as the ideal method of utilizing female employees in post-EEOL Japan. Although only a few companies used this type of system, it is 'ideal' type as same as Japanese management system was; many Japanese companies used a human resource management that was essentially the same and actually based on gender, explicitly or implicitly.

Under the course-based management system, men who graduated from college[3] were hired for *sogo-shoku*. In contrast, most women were hired for *ippan-shoku* even if they were college graduates. In other words, the *ippan-shoku* course was the default course in the human resource management system for female employees (Senda 2001). Very few women who graduated from prestigious colleges were hired for *sogo-shoku*. In fact, under the course-based management system, 80 % of women were in *ippan-shoku* positions in 1993; only 6 % were in *sogo-shoku* positions (Table 4.1).

[2]The targets of the survey were 2310 listed companies from the securities exchanges in Tokyo, Osaka, and Nagoya. The valid respondents were 1042 companies; the valid response rate was 45.1 %.

[3]Male high-school graduates were treated differently from male college graduates. They were allocated jobs that were more similar to those of female workers at the beginning if they were hired as white collar workers or they were hired as blue collar workers. Anyway, they were guaranteed lifelong employment (Nomura 2007). They were classified into *ippan-shoku* if the two classifications of employees were adopted as I've heard from a survey subject in study 2 in Chap. 4.

The details of the system differed by company; in addition to the typical classifications of *sogo-shoku* and *ippan-shoku*, some companies used classifications such as semi-*sogo-shoku* and *senmon-shoku* (a hybrid between *sogo-shoku* and *ippan-shoku*) (Table 4.1).

Semi-*sogo-shoku* and *senmon-shoku* were more similar to *ippan-shoku* than *sogo-shoku* in the sense that they engaged in a limited range of work and had no possibility of job transfers that required relocation. These positions had two purposes. First, these positions were used as a treatment for new female college graduates. Companies required those women to work at a slightly higher level from the beginning, compared to women who graduated from high school or two-year college. In this case, the semi-*sogo-shoku* and *senmon-shoku* courses explicitly indicated the company's requirements. Another purpose was to use these courses as route for promotion from *ippan-shoku*. The ceiling of *ippan-shoku* was set to be within a given set of responsibilities. If women were to continue working after reaching this ceiling, it was beneficial for their career development, as well as for the company, to allow them to be in charge of more difficult tasks, rather than continuing to have them perform the same level of work.

Note that *senmon-shoku* course had existed before the course-based management system was introduced, while semi-*sogo-shoku* course was mainly developed as a treatment for female employees. The *senmon-shoku* course had already been introduced as a treatment for middle-aged non-managerial man (Watanabe 1995). In this way, the ratio occupied by women in *senmon-shoku* course was lower than that of semi-*sogo-shoku* course (Table 4.1).

Companies were reluctant to utilize women based on the following reasons: there were not many female workers with advanced skills, their length of service was short, and they were not their family's main breadwinners (Rodoshinbunsha 2007). The companies claimed that it was not that they discriminated by gender, but rather that the number of women who qualified happened to be small when they screened workers using reasonable criteria, such as skills, years of service, and so on. This kind of reasoning was deemed to have provided a legitimate legal basis until the revision of the EEOL in 2007 prohibited indirect discrimination.[4]

4.4 The New Way of Working Among Women in the 1960s Cohort

The 1960s cohort began to enter the labour market after graduating from high school in the late 1980s. It was around that time that companies began introducing the course-based management system. Women who graduated and became

[4]However, also note that the 2007 revision of the EEOL did not effectively cover all types of indirect discrimination. What is legal and what is illegal is vague. It is uncertain that such companies' claims should be judged as illegal.

employed around this time were likely to be hired under the category of *ippan-shoku* at companies that used the course-based management system. The level of duties that could be assigned to *ippan-shoku* was limited. In most cases, workers reached the ceiling within a given responsibility by the end of an early career.

Meanwhile, since the late 1980s, the Japanese government implemented the EEOL and CCLL in an attempt to create a workplace environment in which women could continue working and be promoted to management positions if we referred to Bolling (2007) and Kasagi (2013) and supposed what they really meant. Under these two opposing trends, both related to utilizing women as a labour force, the 1960s cohort became the first generation of women who were forced to decide, on their own account, between occupational careers and family careers.

As mentioned above, course-based management was created as a loophole against the EEOL, and was intended to continue the previous Japanese human resource management system. Therefore, the company side regarded women in *ippan-shoku* as a temporary labour force, available only for a short period of time, just as before. It is likely that employees had the same attitude when they first became employed.

However, important changes in the way women worked were occurring around this time. Over time, some women in *ippan-shoku* continued working for longer periods of time than expected. For example, in 1996, the average length of service for women in '9 major general trading companies', where women were typically utilized in the *ippan-shoku* course, was 12.4 years (Toyokeizaishinposha 1997), while the overall average for female employees was 8.2 years (*Basic Survey on Wage Structure*). Groups of women who worked for the same company for long periods of time emerged; nevertheless, they did not work in such a way as to balance work and family while having children. Since the rate of maternity leave was pretty low at general trading companies (Senda 1998a), women who did not have children increased the average length of service by continuing to work for longer periods of time.

The emergence of this new way of working was unintended by both companies and the government. For companies, the clerical women who perform the support tasks required of *ippan-shoku* were supposed to be high-turnover human resources who would marry and retire after working for several years, at most. Meanwhile, the government was streamlining systems, such as childcare leave, in order to allow women to balance work and family, and to develop women into *sogo-shoku* who could climb the corporate ladder to managerial positions just like men.

The change in the female workforce that came out of the institutional reform of the 1980s was actually the emergence of a segment of women who continued to extend the length of their service while holding *ippan-shoku* careers—a different way of working from men—without having children or being promoted.

What were the characteristics of career development among these new, long-serving women? What did they think about work and family?

In the following, we will review three studies I conducted during the 1990s and 2000s. Using recorded, real-time observations of working people, we can grasp the real-life atmosphere of these times. This lets us get at the core of the life courses of our targets with so much presence.

4.5 Study 1: University Graduates' Early Career Development

The differences in human resource management may turn into differences in career development and differences in the subjective careers of workers. What kinds of differences will these variations bring?

To investigate these differences, I conducted a semi-structured interview of university graduates' early career experiences in 1994 (Senda 1995). I targeted individuals who graduated from Seminar B of university A in Tokyo one-to-nine years ago (those who were born between 1963 and 1971); 41 individuals cooperated in the study (Table 4.2). The target length of service was decided using Schein's concept of career development stages, in order to capture the 'early career stage' (Schein 1978) as the target of this study. As Schein indicated, individuals move from their early career stage to their middle stage around their 30s; therefore, a

Table 4.2 Attributes of the study subjects

Subjects	Gender	Course	Marital status	Have a child	Change jobs	Number of years from graduation	Year of birth
<1>	F	*Senmon-shoku*	Married	Yes	Yes	9	1963
<2>	M	*Sogo-shoku*	Married	Yes	No	8	1964
<3>	F	*Senmon-shoku*	Married	Yes	Yes	8	1964
<4>	F	*Sogo-shoku*	Married	No	No	7	1965
<5>	M	*Sogo-shoku*	Married	No	No	7	1965
<6>	F	*Senmon-shoku*	Married	No	Yes	7	1965
<7>	M	*Sogo-shoku*	Married	Yes	No	7	1965
<8>	F	*Sogo-shoku*	Married	No	No	6	1966
<9>	F	*Sogo-shoku*	Married	No	No	4	1968
<10>	M	*Sogo-shoku*	Married	Yes	No	3	1969
<11>	F	*Ippan-shoku*	Single	No	No	8	1964
<12>	M	*Sogo-shoku*	Single	No	Yes	8	1964
<13>	F	*Ippan-shoku*	Single	No	No	8	1964
<14>	M	*Sogo-shoku*	Single	No	No	8	1964
<15>	M	*Sogo-shoku*	Single	No	No	7	1965
<16>	M	*Sogo-shoku*	Single	No	No	7	1965
<17>	M	*Sogo-shoku*	Single	No	No	6	1966
<18>	F	*Sogo-shoku*	Single	No	No	6	1966
<19>	M	*Sogo-shoku*	Single	No	No	6	1966
<20>	F	*Sogo-shoku*	Single	No	No	5	1967

(continued)

Table 4.2 (continued)

Subjects	Gender	Course	Marital status	Have a child	Change jobs	Number of years from graduation	Year of birth
<21>	F	*Ippan-shoku*	Single	No	No	5	1967
<22>	M	*Sogo-shoku*	Single	No	No	4	1968
<23>	M	*Sogo-shoku*	Single	No	No	4	1968
<24>	F	*Sogo-shoku*	Single	No	Yes	4	1968
<25>	F	*Sogo-shoku*	Single	No	No	4	1968
<26>	M	*Sogo-shoku*	Single	No	No	3	1969
<27>	M	*Sogo-shoku*	Single	No	No	3	1969
<28>	F	*Sogo-shoku*	Single	No	No	3	1969
<29>	F	*Sogo-shoku*	Single	No	No	3	1969
<30>	F	*Sogo-shoku*	Single	No	No	2	1970
<31>	M	*Sogo-shoku*	Single	No	No	2	1970
<32>	F	*Ippan-shoku*	Single	No	No	2	1970
<33>	F	*Sogo-shoku*	Single	No	No	2	1970
<34>	F	*Sogo-shoku*	Single	No	No	2	1970
<35>	M	*Sogo-shoku*	Single	No	No	2	1970
<36>	M	*Sogo-shoku*	Single	No	No	2	1970
<37>	M	*Sogo-shoku*	Single	No	Yes	2	1970
<38>	F	*Sogo-shoku*	Single	No	No	2	1970
<39>	M	*Sogo-shoku*	Single	No	No	2	1970
<40>	F	*Sogo-shoku*	Single	No	No	1	1970
<41>	F	*Sogo-shoku*	Single	No	No	1	1971

nine-year length of service was regarded as the end of the target stage. Among the study subjects were 4 women in *ippan-shoku*, 3 women in *senmon-shoku* (a hybrid between *sogo-shoku* and *ippan-shoku*), 15 women in *sogo-shoku* (including workers without a course category), and 19 men. In the following analysis, I integrated *ippan-shoku* and *senmon-shoku* into *ippan-shoku*. Among the study subjects, 31 were single and 10 were married. Five individuals had children. Of the 41 study subjects, 29, the equivalent of 70 %, were born in the 1960s. It can be said that this study captured the characteristics of the 1960s cohort.

4.5.1 The Career Development Process

The career development process was extracted from interviews with the study subjects. Some 'phases' that were found to be common across interviewees were identified through an in-depth reading of the interview transcripts. The arrangement of phases and the timings with which they were experienced were different

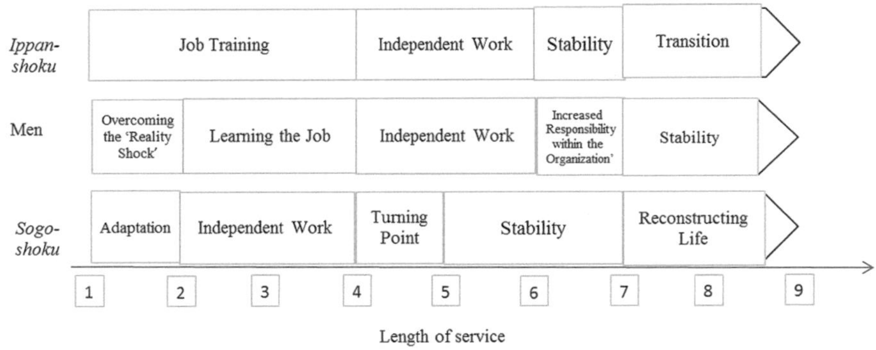

Fig. 4.2 Phases in early careers

among people in different courses. Figure 4.2 presents brief diagrams of the early-stage career development by course. Tables 4.3, 4.4 and 4.5 provide descriptions of the details. The tables carry comments from my interviews without identifying the speaker, in accordance with the requests of some of the interviewees to remain anonymous in the data.

The early career development for *ippan-shoku* (details in Table 4.3) can be summarised as follows: the early career development stage consists of four sub-stages, which can be named the 'job-training phase', 'independent work phase', 'stabilised phase', and 'transition phase'.

The 'job-training phase' is the period in which an individual who knew nothing about the job becomes somewhat capable of performing all aspects of their job without the assistance of others. The period lasted from the first to third year after joining the company.

The 'independent work phase' was a period in which the employee became capable of effortlessly performing the job. Having become familiar with work and starting to feel that life has become easier, they tried to enrich their lives by taking classes, and so on. This period lasted from the fourth to fifth year after they began working.

The 'stabilised phase' is the period in which the employee feels that their work is rewarding and felt pleasure in demonstrating capabilities at work. The sixth year after the start of work was considered such a period. However, there was a limit to the extent of work that an employee on the *ippan-shoku* course can be in charge of.

Once in the 'transition phase', the employee begins to feel that limitation. They became uncomfortable as they think it will be boring to continue to do the same work in the future, and wonder what they should do now. This period is considered to take place from the seventh year on after starting work.

This is a summary of the *ippan-shoku* women's early-stage career development. We will compare this to the career development of men, and then to that of *sogo-shoku* women.

Women in *ippan-shoku* did not experience the 'reality shock' like men did. Since men began their occupational life on the premise that they would continue

Table 4.3 The early career development of women in *Ippan-shoku* course

Phase	Developmental task	Period	Typical comments
Job training	Learning the job	First one to three years of employment	'I think work is fairly interesting'
			'I learned how to perform clerical tasks in the first year. Since then, I'm gradually expanding the range of work that I perform because I have extra time'
			'I cannot help but work hard because everyone around me regards me as "she's already on the third year"'
Independent work	Life becomes easier as one adjusts to work	The fourth and fifth years after the start of work	'I've learned the basics of my entire job. I don't make mistakes as long as I stay alert'
			'The work is becoming easier. Since I still have energy after working all day, I'm taking classes after work'
Stabilised	Demonstrating one's own ability at work	The sixth year after the start of work	'Work responsibility is gradually increasing'
			'I get used to the current job and my occupational life begins to stabilise. Also, I'm thinking of my next occupational career development. These two things are happening in parallel'
Transition	Feeling the limitations of one's position within the organisation and beginning to think about the outlook of one's future career	From the seventh year of employment onwards	'I don't think I can continue doing *ippan-shoku* work at the company much longer. I don't think I can advance my career from here with *ippan-shoku*. I need to start thinking about what I'll do next'
			'The responsibility is becoming too much at work. I'm wondering if this job is worth continue devoting myself in the future'
			'I'll probably be doing the same work up until I turn 30 or so. After that, I don't know'

Table 4.4 The early career development of men

Phase	Developmental task	Period	Typical comments
Overcoming the 'reality shock'	Overcoming the shock of discovering a gap between the reality of employment and the ideal occupation envisioned before starting to work. Adapting oneself to the reality of work life	The first year of employment	'When I was in school, I never really thought about what it meant to work, although I thought I did'
			'When I was in school, I thought about working in an organisation in a way that suits me. The reality is different'
			'They told me "You would never be placed in that department." But I was assigned to the department that I knew I didn't want to be assigned to even before I joined the company'
			'The company only shows the good side before you join, so I thought I would be fine. But the reality is different from what I envisioned'
			'They assigned me a large task from the beginning without any warning'
Job-training	Learning the job	The second to third years after the start of work	'For now, I think I'm going to learn the job'
			'I learned how to manage my tasks'
Independent work	Becoming capable of performing all aspects of the job on their own	The fourth to fifth year after the start of work	'You can't really understand the work until you work at least three years'
			'I'm beginning to see all aspects of my job and understand the meaning of work'
			'As I get used to the company and work, I enjoy being able to perform well at work'.
Assuming responsibility for the organisation	Assuming responsibilities for the organisation. Accepting one's part in the organisation	The sixth year after the start of work	'There is no one else to do the work if I don't'
			'Ultimately, to work is to first do what you are told to do'
			'I'm being swallowed by the company'
			'I'm at the point where the levels of positions are starting to vary. The real competition is starting now'

(continued)

Table 4.4 (continued)

Phase	Developmental task	Period	Typical comments
Stability within the organisation and future dreams coexist	Looking back on the past to gain a sense that one is in the right occupation. Beginning to envision who they want to be in ten years	From the seventh year of employment onwards	'I'm confident in myself now'
			'I've grown in my own way'
			'I think I'm at a milestone'
			'Managing people, rather than directly performing tasks, is becoming my job'
			'Although I have aspirations for another job, I don't think I would change my job'
			'I have become stability-oriented. I don't think I would go elsewhere now'
			'If I were to do something new, I think now is the last chance'
			'Ten years from now, I would like to have achieved something amazing'

Table 4.5 The early career development of women in *Sogo-shoku* course

Phase	Developmental task	Period	Typical comments
Adaptation	Becoming familiar with work	First year of employment	'The first year was physically hard because the work was demanding'
			'The first year was mentally hard because the work was demanding'
Independent work	Becoming capable of performing all aspects of the job	The second to third years after the star of work	'I'm in the process of becoming a fully-qualified person'
			'I would like to continue working in this field'
Turning-point	Looking back on one's occupational career evaluating one's self	The fourth year after the start of work	'Having worked for three years, I've reached a point where I can pause'
			'I've worked for three years, but it was not what I wanted. I found another job'
Stabilised	Applying experience gained on the job	The fifth to sixth years after the start of work	'I'm becoming confident in completing the assigned work on my own at a certain level'
			'I'm finally at the point where I can apply what I have learned so far'

(continued)

Table 4.5 (continued)

Phase	Developmental task	Period	Typical comments
Reconstructing life	Looking back on occupational life and determining the direction of life moving forward	From the seventh year of employment onwards	'I'm at the stage where the levels of promotion begin varying. The real competition is starting now. I'd be lying if I said I didn't care for promotion. I don't want to get behind. But I'm getting so tired that I don't know if I can keep going'
			'Since I'm getting married soon, I'm planning to take marriage as an opportunity to think about what I want to do in the future and what my next step is'
			'I would like to add some qualifications in the future so that I can be reemployed even if I end up quitting work once'
			'I'm thinking about doing something closer to my hobby in order to earn a living'

working for the rest of their life, they envisioned the way they wished to work on a long-term basis before being employed. They were clear in what work they wanted to do from the beginning, and imagined themselves as energetically handling the work they wished to do. However, the reality turned out to be different; it was simply not realistic to think that new hires could handle new jobs one after the other. Instead, they had to start out as assistants. They were not placed in the departments of their choice. Yet, because they have to continue working their whole lives, men adapted themselves to their actual work life.

Ippan-shoku women only planned to work for a short period of time, stating that 'as a starter, I'll work for three years', before becoming employed. Since they were only going to work for a short period of time, they focused on spending their time at a comfortable workplace rather than focusing on the type of work they wanted to do. Since they accepted all tasks they were assigned to do while thinking 'this is the way it is', there was no reality shock, as long as the workplace was comfortable.

Although the timing for the 'independent work phase' was almost the same for both women in *ippan-shoku* and men, the details were different. Those in *ippan-shoku* strived to enrich their private lives by taking classes, and engaging in similar activities once they became competent enough to perform their job with ease. Their reasoning was that 'I should enjoy my time while I'm single without responsibilities because I won't have time for myself once I get married and become tied to housework'. For men, becoming competent enough to perform their job on their own and beginning to enjoy the results produced by their work led to the next step 'increased responsibility in the organisation'. Therefore, men worked more diligently than ever, driven by the sense of mission that 'if not me, who will do the work?'

The final sub-stage of their early careers also differed between women in *ippan-shoku* and men. There was a limit to the extent to the level of work that could be assigned to those in *ippan-shoku*. Once in the last sub-stage of their early career, the 'transition phase', those in *ippan-shoku* began to keenly feel this limit. They felt restless, thinking 'I will probably continue working because I have no plan to get married, but it will probably be boring to continue doing the same job. What should I do from now on?' The final sub-stage of the early career for men was the 'phase in which their stability in the organisation and future dreams coexist'. They looked back over the past and gained a sense of being in the right profession. They began thinking about who they want to be in ten years. They felt they had grown in their own way over time, and were more confident in themselves. The sense of being in the right profession oriented them towards stability; they now planned to continue working for the same company. Going forward, their level of work should continue to increase, and they will find the new ambition needed to accomplish something amazing by the end of the next ten years.

Next, we compare *Ippan-shoku* and *Sogo-shoku* women. *Sogo-shoku* women experienced a different pattern in their early career.

Women in *sogo-shoku* experienced a hard day's work, both mentally and physically, when starting their career. Those in *ippan-shoku* did not experience such hard days. Whereas the first phase continued for three years for those in *ippan-shoku,* it was only one year for those in *sogo-shoku*. *Ippan-shoku* were given three years to learn how to handle work on their own, while *sogo-shoku* were given just one year.

During their fourth year in the workplace, both the *ippan-shoku* and *sogo-shoku* entered into a new phase. However, the ways in which they entered differed. For *ippan-shoku,* it was an 'independent work phase' while for *sogo-shoku*, it was a 'turning point phase'. *Ippan-shoku* enjoyed both work and private activities, based on their feeling capable in their daily work life. They thought it would be good for them to continue on their current path. *Sogo-shoku* women also felt a sense of accomplishment for what they had done; however, this sense of accomplishment did not always make them believe that they were on the right path. Some of them changed jobs.

After that phase, both the *ippan-shoku* and *sogo-shoku* entered into the 'stabilised phase', although the details were different. During this phase, *ippan-shoku* women thought 'I get used to the current job and my occupational life begins to stabilise but work responsibility is gradually increasing', while *sogo-shoku* women thought that they finally reached the point at which they could effectively handle their work in their own way.

The last phases of their early career shared some similarities. Both *ippan-shoku* and *sogo-shoku* came to a point where they hesitated to continue their careers with their current company. For *ippan-shoku,* this hesitation was due to the limits to their work responsibility, which caused them to have a negative view of their prospect for development in the position they currently held. For *sogo-shoku*, some became tired of the competition for promotions, while others just wanted to shift their career in a direction that would fit their interests.

4.5.2 Attitude Towards Work

The tasks performed by women in *ippan-shoku* are characterized by the fact that, although they are not conducting simple clerical work and are required to make judgments, their responsibilities are not large. The interview data show that there was a strong tendency to consider the work as fulfilling and fun. Women in *ippan-shoku* considered their work as a means to support themselves while being single. Therefore, they focused on their work conditions.

The thought processes of women in *sogo-shoku* are in contrast to this. For them, work was a means of expressing themselves. 'I learned the job' meant that they became capable of performing tasks; it did not include the ability to effectively handle the human relations in the organisation. As their work responsibility increased, they began to wonder whether working in that organisation was worth the effort. They thought that they would not mind doing volunteer work, as long as they could apply themselves, because they supposed that there would be no competition among co-workers and that they engage in more substantial work that would match their abilities.

The male interviewees expressed different attitudes towards work. For men, 'I learned the job' meant that not only did they master how to apply themselves in the organisation, but they also learned how to obtain buy-in from the organisation by managing the people around them. The idea was that 'you are foremost expected to thoroughly take care of the tasks assigned by the company because you are a salaried employee'. One interviewee commented that 'you have to work to support yourself. In order to work, it's better if you feel fulfilment. If you have to work anyway, it's better to do your best to achieve results and improve yourself'. Men had a tendency to try to self-actualise by executing the tasks assigned to them. Another interviewee commented that 'work is a good way to express yourself in order to make your dream of accomplishing something big come true'. Their lives were thus centred on work.

4.5.3 Attitude Towards Family

Most women in *ippan-shoku* felt that there was a limit to the level of work they were assigned. However, they had assumed that they would quit their job for marriage or childbirth, before their level of work reached that limit. Therefore, they did not complain that there was a limit to the level of work they would receive.

They wanted to prioritise housework and childcare over work. In particular, they wanted to focus on raising children. They were so family-oriented. Most of the interviewees said that they would not work while raising a child, and considered becoming seeking employment once their child became old enough. They considered part-time jobs to be desirable when seeking reemployment.

As for women in *sogo-shoku*, they felt anxiety toward a new domain of life—family life—that would appear when they married. While work was also important, they felt they had the responsibility of running the family life. In particular, they felt they had the responsibility of raising children. They felt that they had an obligation to choose the family-oriented life. At the same time, they had concerns about whether they could balance a family-oriented life with the occupational life that would become more demanding as the level of expectations at work increased.

Due to the lack of flexible schedules, 11 of the 15 of *sogo-shoku* women felt it was not possible to continue working at the company after they married. They planned to look for a job with a flexible schedule once they were married, because it was impossible to keep the same job they had before marriage, even though they wanted to continue working after marriage.

For men, home was an oasis and a place where housework services were provided. They felt they had a responsibility to support their families. They felt an obligation to feed their families by working for a company, even if it meant giving up what they wanted to do.

Here, Schein's organizational career development stage model (Schein 1978) will be referred to. Only men safely arrived at the end of the early career stage, where both the employees and employer accepted each other, and where the employees have a positive view of their upcoming career within that organization. Both *ippan-shoku* and *sogo-shoku* reached the same stage; however, they failed to reach the mutual acceptance and instead developed a negative attitude towards their future career with that organization. Referring to Super's life-career rainbow model (1980),[5] anticipating one's role as a homemaker differently affected employees' prospects for career development within their organization among women *ippan-shoku*, women *sogo-shoku*, and men.

4.6 Study 2: Survey of Experienced *Ippan-Shoku* Employees

As seen in Study 1, *ippan-shoku* employees may quit when they marry or have a baby, because they prioritize their family over work. Study 1 also showed that there is an upper limit to the types of jobs that can be given to *ippan-shoku* workers and that, after being with a company for seven years, these women began to feel that they have reached an upper limit and started thinking about what to do next.

Study 2 showed how a sample of long-term *ippan-shoku* employees overcame those limitations and continued working. Between 1999 and 2000, I conducted a series of semi-structured interviews among women who were in the *ippan-shoku* course for five or more years (Senda and Ouchi 2002). Fifty interviewees were selected using snow-ball sampling. The breakdown of birth years among the study

[5]In his model, we perform six roles (child, student, leisurite, citizen, worker, and homemaker) during our life course. He stated that the role of worker began in one's mid-20s (this means when one graduates from school) and the role of homemaker subsequently appears in one's late-20s (a little after one begins to work).

subjects was as follows: 3 individuals were born in the late 1950s, 34 individuals were born in the 1960s, and 13 were born in the early 1970s. The 1960s cohort accounted for 70 % of the survey subjects. I can therefore say that the survey subjects adequately capture the situations of *ippan-shoku* workers born into the 1960s cohort. The survey subjects included 19 single individuals and 31 married individuals. Eleven of them had children, and 40 individuals remained at their first job while 10 quit their first job. Among those 10 individuals, 4 had stopped working at the time of the survey and 6 had changed jobs (Table 4.6).

In the following section, comments from the survey subjects will be quoted. Speakers are identified using the survey subject ID (<1> through <50>) listed in Table 4.6.

4.6.1 *The Expected Length of Service for* Ippan-Shoku *Employees*

The 1960s cohort mainly entered the workplace in the 1980s. At that time, it was common for women to quit working once they married, usually after a few years of starting their job. Even after the EEOL was enacted in the latter half of the 1980s, companies expected their female employees with high-school degrees (*ippan-shoku*) to stay for about five years. The work environment ensured their length of service would be short:

> Everyone felt that (high-school graduate) female employees would keep working for five years at the most, and quit at 23 to get married. When they got to that age, some quit 'to get married' even if they weren't really getting married. There weren't any older women at the company. <41>

In the early 1990s, while most companies generally maintained their traditional view toward the expected length of service for female employees, some companies tried thinking in a new way. For instance, a study subject said the following about one company that maintained the traditional view:

> At the company initiation ceremony, we were told, 'Here, women's work is important to the company's success! Junior college grads! Don't quit in 5 years! University grads! Don't quit in 3 years!' <37>

According to a study subject employed at another company that tried out the new way of thinking:

> A notice was sent around the office saying that it was forbidden to encourage women to quit because they were getting married. <41>

4.6.2 *On the Career Intentions at the Time of Employment*

On the one hand, companies had a 'suitable standard' for deciding what the appropriate length of service for their *ippan-shoku* employees should be. However, what intentions did the women of the 1960s cohort have for their career span during their time of employment? One characteristic was that their outlooks on issues like 'How long will I work?' were diverse. Some women intended to quit when they married, while others did not. Some intended to quit when they had a child, while others intended to continue working even after. Some had not yet decided or did not know when they would quit, or they thought whether they quit would depend on the circumstances.

Only two of the survey participants clearly intended, when they started working, to quit when they married, while another three clearly intended to work until retirement. These women had elected to take the *ippan-shoku* career path because it seemed to be an easier way of balancing work and family compared to the *sogo-shoku* path. However, the vast majority of participants did not have a clear idea of how long they would work. They had vaguely thought that they might quit if they married, or if they had a baby, or that their continuing to work would depend on who they married. These three groups correspond to Hakim's classification of women's lifestyle preferences: Home-centered, work-centered, and adaptive (Hakim 2000).

4.6.3 On the Reasons to Continue to Work

For Study 2, subjects who had five or more years of service were selected. As we have seen, five years was the upper limit for the length of service that companies expected from women. The women in Study 2 exceeded that limit. Organizing their subjective observations on why they continued to work resulted in the following themes.

1. They continued to work because they wanted to

A small number of women had intended, from the day they started, to continue working for their entire lives.

> Through high school it was my dream to get married and devote myself to my husband. In junior college I changed my mind after taking a course in women's studies. Rather than living my life relative to someone else, like 'someone's wife' and 'someone's mother', I started to think I had to live my life relative only to myself. So, although I'd like to get married and have children, I decided to try to work for my whole life. <5>

From the moment this woman started looking for a job, she adopted the strategy of selecting a company that had a record of valuing the work of its female employees. After being hired, she was proactive, for example, in asking for transfers when the work was too demanding or when she thought she was not suited for the work, and so on.

2. They continued to work because they had to

Although few in number, some of the subjects had intended, from the time they were hired, to quit when they married, but they were still working. One participant <42> had the clear intention of quitting 'after working about five years' or, in any case, 'soon'. At the time of the survey, she was still thinking that, if her personal situation made it possible, she would quit. It was because she married later in life

Table 4.6 Occupational careers and family career among the study subjects

Life stage	First job stage	Year of entry	Year of birth	Education	Subject	Years on the job 1	2	3	4	5	6	7	8
Single	Held	1993	1974	H	<1>	—	—	—	●	—	★	P	
		1987	1968	H	<2>	—	○	—	—	☆	—	—	—
		1992	1971	TC	<3>	—	○	○	—	○	—	★	W
		1991	1970	TC	<4>	—	—	—	○	—	—	—	○
		1987	1966	TC	<5>	—	—	—	□	■	—	—	—
		1987	1966	TC	<6>	—	—	■	—	—	—	—	—
		1982	1961	TC	<7>	—	—	—	—	—	—	—	—
		1980	1959	TC	<8>	—	—	—	—	—	—	—	—
		1993	1970	C	<9>	—	—	○	—	—	⇒	■	
		1993	1970	C	<10>	—	—	★	—	—	★	→	
		1987	1964	C	<11>	—	—	—	—	—	—	→	
		1992	1969	C	<12>	—	—	—	—	—	—	—	☆
		1990	1967	C	<13>	—	●	—	●	—	—	—	—
		1990	1967	C	<14>	—	★	—	⇒	—	—	F	—
		1990	1967	C	<15>	①	—	☆	—	①	—	—	—
		1989	1966	C	<16>	—	—	—	★	—	—	—	—
		1989	1966	C	<17>	—	—	⇒	○	—	●	—	—
		1989	1966	C	<18>	—	—	—	—	○	—	—	—
	Quit	1983	1960	V	<19>	—	—	—	—	—	—	D①	—
Married (No child)	Held	1991	1970	TC	<20>	—	—	○	—	—	—	PF	●
		1990	1969	TC	<21>	●	—	—	☆	—	—	—	—
		1989	1968	TC	<22>	①	—	—	∞□	○	—	—	—
		1989	1968	TC	<23>	—	☆	—	—	☆	—	—	—
		1988	1967	TC	<24>	—	—	—	—	—	—	—	—
		1994	1971	C	<25>	—	—	⇒	—	—	→		
		1993	1970	C	<26>	—	—	—	—	—	—	●	
		1993	1970	C	<27>	—	—	—	●	—	—	→	
		1993	1970	C	<28>	—	—	☆	—	—	—	→	
		1993	1970	C	<29>	—	—	⇒	F	P	—	→	
		1990	1967	C	<30>	—	—	—	—	—	—	—	—
		1988	1965	C	<31>	—	—	—	—	—	—	—	—
		1983	1960	C	<32>	—	—	—	—	—	—	—	—
	Quit	1989	1968	TC	<33>	—	○	—	○	—	∞	—	—
		1988	1967	TC	<34>	—	—	N	—	—	—	—	—
		1988	1967	TC	<35>	—	—	—	—	—	—	—	—
		1993	1970	C	<36>	—	—	△	—	●	R	D	
		1989	1966	C	<37>	①	—	—	—	—	—	—	—
		1989	1966	C	<38>	—	—	—	—	—	Pt	—	R
		1988	1965	C	<39>	—	—	○	—	☆	—	—	★
Married (with child)	Held	1990	1971	H	<40>	—	—	—	—	—	—	—	—
		1987	1968	H	<41>	—	—	○	⇒	—		—	—
		1984	1965	H	<42>	—	—	—	—	—	—	—	—
		1989	1968	TC	<43>	①	■	—	—	☆1	—	※	※
		1987	1966	TC	<44>	—	—	—	⇒	—	※	—	—
		1975	1954	TC	<45>	—	—	○	—	—	—	—	—
		1991	1968	C	<46>	—	—	—	—	∫※	○		—
		1990	1967	C	<47>	—	●	○	—	○	—	※	○
		1990	1967	C	<48>	○	—	—	—	☆	—	—	○
	Quit	1989	1968	TC	<49>	—	—	⇒	—	—	■	□	—
		1980	1959	TC	<50>	—	●1	⇒	—	—	○	①	—

(continued)

Table 4.6 (contiuned)

9	10	11	12	13	14	15	16	17	18	19	20	21	22	23	24	25
—	—	—	—	∞												
○																
⇒	—	—	—	→												
⇒	—	∞	□	→												
—	—	—	—	—	—	∞	→									
—	○	●1	—	—	—	—	—	—	★	—	○1					
—	→															
—	→															
—	→															
—	—	→														
—	—	→														
—	—	P●														
—	—	—	—	—	○	①	—	→								
→																
∞	→															
—	—	①□														
☆	○	→														
∞	★	○	→													
→																
—	○	☆														
—	—	—	—	—	—	—	→									
R	D	→														
R	D	—	→													
—	—	—	R													
☆	①N	→														
—	○	N	→													
※	→															
—	—	※	—	→												
—	—	—	—	—	※	∫										
∬	—	→														
—	⇒	—	—	⇒P												
△	—	—	—	—	—	—	—	—	—	—	—	—	∞	—	○	△
※																
—	→															
○	※															
∞	—	R														
—	—	—	F	—		※	∫R									

◀ Transfer at the convenience of the company: ○ Intra-division, ● Inter-division; Transfer to a subsidiary company: △ Intra-division, ▲ Inter-division; Transfer hoped by employee: ☆ Intra-division, ★Inter-division; Transfer for career development: □ Intra-division, ■ Inter-division; Job enlargement: ⇒ Intra-division; Transfer accompanying childrearing: ʃ Intra-division, ʃʃ Inter-division
Education; *C* college, *T C* two-year college, *V* vocational school, *H* high school
Promotions; ∞ promoted, *P* passed a course-change test, *F* failed a course-change test, *W* waiting for the result of a course-change test
Transfer to the section once allocated; ① and 1 denote the same section
Change in employment; *R* resigned, *N* new job, *D* dispatched worker, *Pt* part-time worker
※ Child care leave
The *solid line* connects years of marriage. The *dotted line* connects the years related to the birth of their first child (including expectations)

that she had to continue working. When, in her 14th year of work, she married, her husband asked her to continue working in order to help the family budget, and so she continued working. Then, when she became pregnant, her husband again asked her to keep working in order to help support their family. She thought that 'On my husband's salary alone we would barely get by, but if we both work we have a little to spare'. She worked purely because she had to for her family. As she thought about what to do next, and about the direction of her career, she wanted to have one more child, and thought that she would probably continue working even after the second child was born. However, that view was completely contingent on her 'having to work to make ends meet'.

3. 'It just happened'/'I just got carried along'

The overwhelming majority of the subjects of this survey began working with only vague ideas about the future, such as, for example: 'I haven't decided', 'I don't know how long I will work', and 'It depends'. Once they actually started to work, they found the work interesting, and because the social norms for what was a marriageable age had weakened and company atmospheres had become more accepting of women who did not quit when they married, these women started to think that they might not quit because of marriage after all. Thus, when they actually did get married, they continued working.

There were three reasons the subjects found their work interesting. The first was the depth of *ippan-shoku* work:

> I enjoy clerical work. I feel motivated. For example, the order system can get jammed if the entry timing for the sales vouchers is off. When that happens, I work with someone from the technology department to fix how the vouchers get processed. By finding ways to better organize the filing so it is easy to refer to later, I can make work more efficient. Because I end up knowing a lot about how our clients' offices work, when I have to contact a client for something, I know enough to avoid Mr. X, who is so difficult to deal with, and ask for Mr. Y. <37>

The second reason was due to transfers linked to developing their skills. Subject <3> requested a transfer because her quotas were difficult to meet and, with her manager's recommendation, she transferred to the training department. After two months of training, she became responsible for the training of new employees.

I feel motivated in my current job. I've done a few different jobs, and this is the first time I've felt motivated. As an instructor in training, the trainees rely on me and admire me. Trainees have sometimes told me 'I'd like to become a trainer someday!' and sometimes after a training program, I get a call from a trainee saying '*Sensei!* (Professor!) I don't know how to process this work, so would it be possible for you to help me?!' It's not that I know how to do everything in this company, but because I'm relied on in that way, rather than saying 'I don't know', I learn how to do it. I'd love to do even more of this work. <3>

The third reason for employees choosing to remain at their jobs was the expansion of their responsibilities to a degree that they then overlapped with those of the *sogo-shoku* employees.

In the past when imported goods were damaged in transit, one of the men in the office negotiated with the insurance company, but I started taking care of that myself. The other party acknowledged me as the person to negotiate with and my boss also told me to go right ahead. When something is damaged, you go out and have a look at it and negotiate with the insurance company, telling them how much damage there was and how much compensation we want for it. Depending how much compensation we get, we can make or lose money on the deal. Because our company and the insurance company have competing interests, a third-party institution makes an appraisal of the damage. I found that I was able to negotiate with the auditor to get an assessment in our favor by telling him, 'if we don't get a little more from the insurance, we'll be stuck with a loss, so please help me out!' When I managed to get an agreement with conditions in our favor, I came back to the office and impressed my colleagues by showing off how much compensation I got. I enjoyed that! <8>

Notwithstanding the fact that quitting in order to marry has become less frequent, these women generally resisted the idea of continuing to work after having a baby. Of the 32 study participants who worked but did not have children (19 single, 13 married without children), there were only 6 women who intended to continue working even after giving birth.

However, looking at the 11 women who actually had a baby, their decisions to continue to work were determined by their circumstances. They elected to continue working because their work experiences were motivating, because they were in environments that were supportive of their continued employment, and because husbands who encouraged them to continue working. Of the 11 women with children, 9 were still working (one woman left after returning from childcare leave and one woman was quitting the job before childbearing).

When all of these women started working, they were unsure of how long they would stay at work, either because they had not yet decided, did not know, or thought it would depend on their circumstances. The following are examples of the reasons they gave for continuing to work:

My husband told me he wanted me to keep working and with the times as they are, he could lose his job, so it's better if I work, as well, as insurance just in case. <42>

My female colleagues told me that it would be such a waste to do anything like throw away the stability of having the status of regular employee without even trying to see if I could manage both, so I decided to try it for now. I can always quit (while once I quit, I barely get re-hired as a regular employee). <43>

Once you quit it's hard to get re-hired as a regular employee. It would be such a waste to throw away that status without making any attempt to keep it. <44>

It would be such a waste to throw away the career I've built over all this time. <46>

4.6.4 The 'High-Performing Ippan-Shoku': *Advantages and Bottlenecks*

These women were 'high-performing *ippan-shoku*', as perceived by themselves as well as by their managers and colleagues. They had developed themselves by gradually expanding the types of work they were capable of doing without ever feeling overburdened.

> I'm happy I built my career by first being an assistant, and after I got used to that, while staying within my abilities, by gradually expanding the breadth of my job. Because you're a 'veteran' after five years, now they keep on giving me more to do. <12>

The advantages of being a high-performing *ippan-shoku* were that these women, while able to feel some level of motivation for their work, did not bear the ultimate responsibility for it (that responsibility fell to the *sogo-shoku* or their managers) and that they could keep their work within reasonable limits, which allowed them to take care of their personal lives.

> In any case, as an *ippan-shoku* worker you are limited as to what types of work you can do and whether you work hard or not has no effect on your evaluation. If you can accept it for what it is, being an *ippan-shoku* worker is a comfortable job to have. <6>

> *Ippan-shoku* responsibilities are lighter, which I find easier. I want to be in a comfortable job. A *sogo-shoku* has to work at overcapacity and tough it out. As an *ippan-shoku*, you can work at your own pace and not over-do it and, you can take good care of your personal life. <12>

However, being a high-performing *ippan-shoku* did not entail only good things. They kept themselves apart from the real challenges of the business because, as useful as their experience may have been, even though they did not work as hard as the *sogo-shoku* employees, they felt that they were not seen as equal in ability, and that their skills were not seen to be of value outside of their departments.

> I am feeling the limitations of being an *ippan-shoku* worker. Because my manager is a proactive user of his *ippan-shoku* staff, I could probably take better advantage of opportunities to improve myself. On the other hand, *ippan-shoku* workers are appreciated for competencies related to their personalities (like being diligent), and I'd like to do a job that makes use of my ability to think. I've had enough of *ippan-shoku* work and am wondering if doing a different job wouldn't be good for me. But then, although my skills are fine for my current workplace, they aren't good enough be an asset if I tried to change jobs. <12>

4.6.5 Work Precedence in the Life Courses

As indicated in Chap. 3, the women in the 1950s cohort worked while 'waiting to get married'. Leaving work to marry was an established path, an early endpoint that was already set at the beginning of a woman's occupational career. Women's working lives were a so-called 'preparation' for marriage. However, by the time that the 1960s cohort had entered the workplace, the social climate had changed. It was recommended for 'even' women to work. As before, marriage and children were deciding factors when women thought about their future, but it became possible to 'first, try working, then think about it'.

In the course of these women's lives, their working lives took precedence over their family life, even to the extent that it was possible that their family lives could be impacted by the need to accommodate their working lives. Three working subjects (single <6>, married without children <25>, and married with children <45>) made the following comments:

> There was a time when I thought about getting married, but it was too difficult for me to give up the work environment. I just kept working and didn't get married. At work there are a lot of excellent men and I like being able to interact with them every day. I don't think much about the future. For the time being, I intend to continue doing what I'm doing, and I just might work until retirement. There isn't any special reason to quit. There are some things, of course, I don't like about my job, but not enough to quit. I'm also not absolutely set on getting married. There have to be a lot of people like me who keep working because there is no reason to quit, don't you think? <6>

> As I continued to work, I realized that it suited me. Staying home (dedicating myself to housework) wouldn't. <25>

> When I was at home for four months for childcare leave, I realized that staying home (dedicating myself to housework and childcare) didn't suit me. <45>

4.6.6 Liberation from the Curse of Being a Homemaker

The women of the 1960s cohort experienced working life before family life, and made choices that affected their life course by comparing how much their commitment to each life sphere suited them. It had already become unprohibited for women not to marry and quit work before a certain age, and to not have children and dedicate their lives to housework and childcare. These women were liberated from the normative curse of having to spend their lives devoted to homemaking.

Although these women were freed from the old norms, living the new life was impossible if their spouses and the people around them were not also freed from those norms. Continuing to work full-time was an effective way of winning the understanding of their peers.

> To have a life in which you are alone with a child everyday all day sounds very stressful to me. I know a number of women who say that compared to that, it' s better to put the child in a nursery during the day while you work, and when you get home from work, you can switch gears and enjoy being back together with your child; and, that's what they do. Before I thought if I had a child I would quit work, but hearing these women's stories, I started to think that I would keep working, too. I was surprised at this change in myself. <21>

> I thought about quitting work when I had a baby, but then, because I don't care for children, I figured it would be better to raise the child while working than to dedicate myself to childcare. <41>

When a woman was working, she could reduce her involvement in housework and childcare by, for example, asking her husband to help or by hiring out help (e.g., putting the child in a nursery).

4.6.7 *The Relationship Between* Ippan-Shoku *Employees with Children and the Workplace*

The phenomenon of women continuing to work after giving birth was no longer limited to those who worked in industries like civil service and education, because some of the ordinary women working for private companies—that is, some *ippan-shoku* workers—had also begun to do so. This study of nine women with children who are/were working for private companies showed that the companies were not prepared to adequately deal with these workers.

They faced two problems. The first problem was with the allocation of work. If a replacement was not temporarily hired for an employee on childcare leave, her colleagues had to pick up her work, which was unfair to them. Furthermore, when she returned from childcare leave, the amount of work to allocate to her was also a problem. One subject quit when her boss was over-considerate and did not give her enough work, because she wondered, 'Is this worth leaving my child at the nursery, crying and screaming because he doesn't want to be separated from me?' The second problem was that some workplaces were simply too busy. When it became natural for everyone to work overtime, being the only person who left work on time was felt to be 'shameful'.

4.6.8 *Drivers of Career Development*

Using the interview data, I identified multiple cases in which tasks that were traditionally performed by *sogo-shoku* workers were transferred to *ippan-shoku* workers. Compared to the regular tasks of the *ippan-shoku*, these are more complex tasks that require making important decisions. This transfer means that *ippan-shoku* workers became responsible of more important work; it can be regarded as being equivalent to the experience of getting more important assignments than before, which is a career development driver noted by Nakamura (1988).

Apart from such transfers, there are also cases in which the subject experienced a job rotation within the office. Some subjects rotated into a related department, while others rotated into an unrelated department. Of these, the cases in which a subject experienced a job rotation to an unrelated department can be regarded as similar to the career development patterns of men in which they gain a wide range of knowledge and skills and expand their network of contacts through experiencing various departments. Higuchi (1991) also pointed out that job rotations encourage female employees to remain with their company.

From this point, we will continue our investigation by quantifying the interview data. First, we will examine the new trends in how companies use *ippan-shoku* workers.

In my interviews, I discovered three types of events that facilitate career development. Seventeen subjects said they had experienced one of the following incidents at least once: an 'inter-division job rotation, which an employee hopes for'

(★ in Table 4.6), an 'inter-division job rotation for career development' (■ in Table 4.6), or 'getting more important assignments' (⇒ in Table 4.6). These three experiences (★, ■, and ⇒) are the career development drivers I discovered. The chances of accepting a career development driver by educational background were as follows: 60 % of high school graduates experienced at least one of these drivers, 33 % of two-year-college and vocational-school graduates experienced at least one driver, and 32 % of college graduates experienced at least one driver.

It is important to note that, with the exception of subject < 44 >, almost all of the subjects were offered these drivers before they were married; this suggests that being single is one of the conditions necessary for receiving such career development opportunities. Conversely, it is possible that such opportunities might not have been available if the subjects were already married. The following statement is a typical representation of this tendency:

> When I was single I had opportunities to improve my skills because I was continually given jobs that were just a little beyond what I could normally do. But, the way my manager assigned me work changed after I got married. For example, he assigns jobs to men without worrying about the overtime it will take, but he holds back and only gives me jobs that can be done without overtime. <22>

4.6.9 Task Allocation Patterns

In the interviews, I asked the subjects how tasks were assigned to their colleagues in the workplace. I collected the latest examples from everyone, including every case at the time of the interview and as many additional cases as possible. Task allocation in the workplace can be classified into the following five types (Senda 2000):

1. Separation Type: The workplace is composed of female *ippan-shoku* staff and a male manager. Tasks are performed by *ippan-shoku* staff and approved by the manager.
2. Secretary Type: The workplace is composed of female *ippan-shoku* staff, male *sogo-shoku* staff, and a male manager. *Ippan-shoku* staff directly report to the manager while also acting as administrative assistants to the manager.
3. Shared Type: The workplace is composed of female *ippan-shoku* staff, male *sogo-shoku* staff, and a male manager. The *Ippan-shoku* staff are paired with the *sogo-shoku* staff. The tasks for a given process are divided between them. For example, the *sogo-shoku* staff go out to get sales orders and the *ippan-shoku* staff process those orders.
4. Management-Assistance Type: The workplace is composed of female *ippan-shoku* staff, male *sogo-shoku* staff, and a male manager. The *ippan-shoku* staff directly report to the manager and also act as junior *sogo-shoku* staff by, for example, accompanying the manager as he attends meetings.
5. Self-Sufficient Type: The workplace is composed of female *ippan-shoku* staff, male *sogo-shoku* staff, and a male manager. All *ippan-shoku* and *sogo-shoku* staff members receive individual assignments and work on their own. The level

Table 4.7 Task allocation for *Ippan-shoku* in the workplace by years of service (%)

Way	Type	1st to 10th year	11th year and on	N
	Separation type	28.4	31.6	27
Traditional	Secretary + shared types	41.3	31.6	41
New	Management assistance + self-sufficient types	24.3	36.8	25
	Total (N)	65	28	93

Table 4.8 Task allocation for *Ippan-shoku* in the workplace by years of service among the pre-EEOL generation (%)

Way	Type	1st to 10th year	11th year and on	N
	Separation type	0	14.3	1
Traditional	Secretary + shared types	55.6	42.9	9
New	Management assistance + self-sufficient types	44.4	28.6	6
	Total (N)	9	7	16

Table 4.9 Task allocation for *Ippan-shoku* in the workplace by years of service among the post-EEOL generation (%)

Way	Type	1st to 10th year	11th year and on	N
	Separation type	26.2	41.7	22
Traditional	Secretary + shared types	46.2	25.0	33
New	Management assistance + self-sufficient types	27.7	33.3	22
	Total (N)	56	21	77

of the allocated task varies by course. For example, when allocating a task, the *ippan-shoku* workers will be in charge of products with minimal price fluctuations, while the *sogo-shoku* workers will handle products with larger price fluctuations.

Of the above five types, the management-assistance type and the self-sufficient type share similar utilization methods, in which *ippan-shoku* employees are asked to do the same work as junior *sogo-shoku* employees. Here, these two types will be called the 'new' way. The secretary type and shared type are both traditional workplaces in which *ippan-shoku* women and *sogo-shoku* men work together, but they receive clearly different treatment under the two management systems. Here, these two types will be called the 'traditional' way. We combine this pair of workplace-types accordingly in the analysis below. As for 'Separation Type', let that word stand.

The differences in task allocation by years of service and by generation are examined in Tables 4.7, 4.8 and 4.9.

Table 4.7 shows how the employees were utilised, arranged according to the employee's years of service. Those who are utilised as 'traditional' way decrease once they exceed 10 years of service, while those under 'new' way increase after 10 years of service. As the years of service increases, more *ippan-shoku* workers were utilised in a manner similar to that of *sogo-shoku* workers; more 'new' way than 'traditional' way.

I looked at task allocation by generation by separating the generation that started working before the EEOL (the pre-EEOL generation)[6] from the generation that started working after the EEOL (the post-EEOL generation) and comparing them (Tables 4.8 and 4.9). There was no pre-EEOL generation individual who was classified under 'Separation Type' during their first through tenth year of service. In the post-EEOL generation, more than a quarter of the survey subjects fell into this category.

The percentage of 'traditional' way was smaller in the post-EEOL generation. The percentage of subjects in the 'new' way was higher in the pre-EEOL generation during the first ten years; however, it was slightly higher in the post-EEOL generation after the eleventh year of service.

Lastly, a trend that is difficult to evaluate will be pointed out. The percentage of the 'Separation Type' pattern was higher in the post-EEOL generation. It is difficult to determine how to evaluate the utilisation of women in a workplace that consists only of female *ippan-shoku* staff and managers, but no *sogo-shoku* staff. It is possible that *ippan-shoku* workers are utilised in a manner similar to junior *sogo-shoku* workers, since *ippan-shoku* workers performed all tasks while managers only verified and approved their work. However, another interpretation may be that they only have *ippan-shoku* workers because those kinds of workplaces do not actually need *sogo-shoku* workers. When viewed this way, I cannot state that companies are utilising *ippan-shoku* workers in the same manner as they would junior *sogo-shoku* workers. It may be that the division of labour by gender has advanced in recent years, with the result that the longer-serving *ippan-shoku* women are beginning to be placed in 'female ghettos'. If that is the case, is that an advantageous or disadvantageous treatment of *ippan-shoku* workers? Making a judgment will be refrained here.

4.7 Study 3: Survey on Special Skills of *Ippan-Shoku* Employees

Study 2 showed how and why long-serving *ippan-shoku* employees continued working. A topic that still needs to be researched is whether *ippan-shoku* workers can offer special skills.

A questionnaire survey on the skills of 814 *ippan-shoku* and *sogo-shoku* workers belonging to a cross-industry networking club and a study group on female labour was conducted in 2002 (101 valid respondents; 12.4 % valid response rate)

---

[6]It should be noted that the number of cases in the pre-EEOL generation was not large.

(Senda 2003). Of those respondents, 96 were regular employees (95.1 %). The average length of service among the regular employees was 17.7 years. There were 53 females and 47 males, with one respondent whose gender was unknown. As for their marital status, about half of the respondents were single, a little over 10 % were married without children, and close to 40 % were married with children.

Based on the survey year and the average length of service among the respondents, it was estimated that 1984 was the average year in which the respondents started working. The average birth year was 1961, if the respondent was a college graduate, and 1965, if the respondent was a high school graduate. Therefore, the respondents displayed the characteristics of the 1960s cohort.

Skills were measured in terms of how well the respondent could handle tasks in their assigned workplace based on the following five criteria: (1) the individual can handle the task on her/his own, (2) the individual can teach the task to others, (3) the individual can handle troubles that arise while completing the task, (4) the individual can propose a new way of handling the task, and (5) the individual can cover others flexibly when the manpower is not adequate. Items (1) through (4) were created based on Koike (1997), and item (5) was created from Senda (1998b). The skill level was measured on a 5-point scale ranging from 'not capable at all' to 'completely capable'.

A difference existed between the groups only for task (5) ('cover others flexibly when the manpower is not adequate'). The percentage of respondents who said they would cover others was high among *ippan-shoku* workers (Table 4.10). This is the special skill of *ippan-shoku* workers.

As Ishida (1999) noted, allocating tasks to employees is not strictly handled in Japanese companies. While it is roughly determined who handles what task, any available individual must handle tasks in emergencies. Workplaces need workers who can play such a role.

Table 4.10 Skill comparison between courses

Course		Handle them without help	Teach them to others	Handle problems	Propose new ways of handling	Cover others flexibly when the manpower is not adequate
Ippan-shoku	Mean	3.75	3.83	4.00	3.75	*4.33*
	S.D.	0.87	0.83	0.85	0.97	*0.65*
	N	12	12	12	12	*12*
Sogo-shoku	Mean	3.86	3.77	3.82	3.86	*3.64*
	S.D.	0.64	0.69	0.59	0.83	*0.79*
	N	22	22	22	22	*22*
Not under course-based system	Mean	3.78	3.67	3.70	3.57	*3.90*
	S.D.	0.90	0.90	0.89	0.83	*0.75*
	N	60	60	60	60	*60*
	Fscale	0.09	0.27	0.72	1.06	*3.36*
	P	0.91	0.77	0.49	0.35	*0.04*

The above results indicate that such irregular tasks are often assigned to *ippan-shoku* women. Such a practice tends to occur because women in the *ippan-shoku* course have worked in a given workplace for a long time without rotating jobs. This is an advantage they have over *sogo-shoku* employees in their workplace, who have less experience in a given workplace because they develop their career through rotating jobs across various workplaces. Thus, *ippan-shoku* workers often become the 'walking dictionary' of the workplace, understanding the overall business that occurs there. When required, they are capable of improvising in order to handle tasks that are not their own. This capability makes them indispensable in their workplace. However, companies are apt to underestimate this ability, which is unique to long-serving *ippan-shoku* employees.

The studies of female clerical workers in Japan have a tendency to describe the deadlock they face in their career (Konno 1996; Ogasawara1998). These studies suggest that *ippan-shoku* employees drive themselves into a corner and isolate themselves, which does not match my findings. This may be because previous research has neglected long-serving employees. To be exact, previous research did not pay attention to the length of service, and regarded female clerical workers as homogeneous. However, there is a difference among those in the early stage of their careers and those in the middle or late stages of their in terms of their skills, job attitude, and so on.

References

Bolling, Patricia. 2007. Policies to support working mothers and children in Japan. In *Political economy of Japan's low fertility*, ed. Rosenbluth, Frances McCall, 131–154. Stanford: Stanford University Press.

Hakim, Chatherine. 2000. *Work-lifestyle Choices in the 21st Century: Preference Theory*. New York: Oxford University Press.

Higuchi, Yoshio. 1991. *Nihon Keizai-to Shugyo Kodo*. Tokyo: Toyo Keizai Shinposha (in Japanese).

Imada, Sachiko, and Shuzo Hirata. 1995. *Howaitokora-no Shoshin Kozo*. Tokyo: Japan Institute of Labor (in Japanese).

Ishida, Hideo. 1999. *Kokusai Keiei-to Howaitokara*. Tokyo: Chuo Keizaisha (in Japanese).

Japan Institution of Workers' Evolution (21-seiki Shokugyo Zaidan). 1994. *Shinki Gakusotsu Saiyo Naitei-to Chosa Kekka Hokokusho* (in Japanese).

Kasagi, Eri. 2013. Kazoku keisei-to ho (Family formation and law). *Nihon Rodo Kenkyu Zassi (The Monthly Journal of the Japan Institute of Labour)* 638: 53–65 (in Japanese).

Kimoto, Kimiko. 2004. Kazoku-to kigyoshakai: Rekishiteki kosatsu. In *Henbosuru Kigyoshakai Nihon (Changing Japan's Rregime: Company-centered Society)*, ed. Watanabe Osamu, 229–340. Tokyo: Junposha (in Japanese).

Koike, Kazuo. 1997. *Nihonkigyo-no Jinzai Keisei: Fukakujitsusei-ni Taishosurutame-no Nouhau*. Tokyo: Chuo Koron Shinposha (in Japanese).

Komagawa, Tomoko. 2013. Bunsekitaisho-to siteno josei jimurodosha-to kyaria (Conducting research on women clerks and careers). *Hokkaido-daigaku Daigakuin Kyoikugaku Kenkyusho Kiyo* 119: 139–154 (in Japanese).

Komagawa, Tomoko. 2014. Seibetsu shokumu bunri-to kyaria keisei-ni okeru danjosa (Job segregation and career gap by gender in bank clerks). *Nihon Rodo Kenkyu Zassi (The Monthly Journal of the Japan Institute of Labour)* 648: 48–59 (in Japanese).

Konno, Minako. 1996. Negotiating gender in uncertainty: A mechanism of women's marginalization in the Japanese workplace. *International Journal of Japanese Sociology* 5(1): 23–40.

Nakamura, Megumi. 1988. Ote supa-ni okeru josei kanrishokusha, senmonshokusha: Shigoto keiken-to kyaria. In *Shokuba-no Kyaria Uman*, eds. Kazuo Koike, and Yasunobu Tomita, 12–37. Tokyo: Toyo Keizai Shinposha (in Japanese).

Nomura, Masami. 2007. *Nihonteki Koyo Kanko: Zentaizo Kochiku-no Kokoromi*. Kyoto: Minerva Shobo (in Japanese).

Ogasawara, Yuko. 1998. *Office ladies and salaried men: power, gender, and work in Japanese Companies*. Berkeley: University of California Press.

Osawa, Mari. 1993. *Kigyo Chushin Shakai-wo Koete: Gendai Nihon-wo Jenda-de Yomu*. Tokyo: Jijitsushinsha (in Japanese).

Rodoshinbunsha. 2007. *Wakariyasui Kaitei Koyou Kikai Kintouhou*. Tokyo: Rodoshinbunsha (in Japanese).

Saito, Osamu. 2013. Dansei kaseginushi moderu-no rekishiteki hensen (Historical origins of the breadwinner household model). *Nihon Rodo Kenkyu Zassi (The Monthly Journal of the Japan Institute of Labour)* 638: 4–16 (in Japanese).

Schein, Edgar H. 1978. *Career dynamics: matching individual and organizational needs*. Reading: Addison-Wesley.

Senda, Yukiko. 1995. *Daisotsusha-no Shoki Kyaria Hattatsu*. Tokyo: Tokyo Josei Zaidan (in Japanese).

Senda, Yukiko. 1998a. Josei jugyoin katsuyo-wo toraeru futatsu-no jigen (Two dimensions of utilization of women employees in companies: Different tendencies among the tertiary industries). *Keiei Kodo Kagaku (Japanese Journal of Administrative Science)* 12(2): 113–124 (in Japanese).

Senda, Yukiko. 1998b. Shosha-ni okeru ippan-shoku-no kyaria: 'Ippan-shoku = tankigata koyo' tsunen-eno hansho. *Sangyo Soshiki Shinri Gakkai Dai 14-kai Taikai Kenkyu Hokoku Ronbunshu*: 181–183 (in Japanese).

Senda, Yukiko. 2000. Jyosei ippan-shoku-no kyaria keisei: Sono-sokushin yoin-to genkai. *Jyosei Rodo Kenkyu* 38: 96–102 (in Japanese).

Senda, Yukiko. 2001. Kosu-betsu koyou kanri-to jenda: Tayosei-wo ikasu. In *Jenda Manegimento: 21-seikigata Danjo Kyoso Kigyo-ni Mukete (Gender Management)*, ed. Yoko Sano, Masamitsu Shimane, and Sumito Shino, 236–265. Tokyo: Toyo Keizai Shinposha (in Japanese).

Senda, Yukiko. 2003. Hi-koa jugyoin-no shakaiteki seiryoku kakutoku-ni okeru komyunikeshon-no koka (The effect of communication over non-core employees' gaining social power). *Tetsugaku (Keio University)* 110: 169–197 (in Japanese).

Senda, Yukiko, and Akiko Ouchi. 2002. Josei seiki jugyoin-no kyaria keisei-no tayose: Kosu betsu koyo kanrii seido-wo tegakari toshite (Career development of female employees: Comparative study of *sogo-shoku* and *ippan-shoku*). *Soshiki Kagaku (Organizational Science)* 36(1): 95–107 (in Japanese).

Super, D.E. 1980. A life-span, life-space approach to career development. *Journal of Vocational Behavior* 16: 282–298.

Tachibanaki Toshiaki (Translated by Mary E. Foster). 2010. *The new paradox for Japanese women: Greater choice, greater inequality (LTCB International Library selection, no. 26)*. Tokyo: LTCB International Library Foundation.

Toyokeizaishinposha. 1997. *Kaisha-shikiho Josigakusei Shushokuban '98*. Tokyo: Toyo Keizai Shinposha (in Japanese).

Watanabe, Takashi. 1995. *Kosu-betsu Koyo Kanri-to Josei Rodo: Danjo Kyodo Sankaku-wo Mezashite*. Tokyo: Chuokeizaisha (in Japanese).

Yashiro, Atsushi. 1995. *Daikigyo Howaitokara-no Kyaria: Ido-to Shoshin-no Bunseki*. Tokyo: Japan Institute of Labour (in Japanese).

Chapter 5
The Work-Family Interface: Balancing on a Knife's Edge

Abstract The author conducted semi-structured interviews of 10 couples in which both spouses worked full-time jobs in the Tokyo Metropolitan Area and at least one spouse took childcare leave. The subjects were born in the 1960s and early 1970s. The results show how difficult it was to continue working full-time while raising a child, how they coped with this difficulty, how childcare leave and the childcare-break system helped them, and how they changed through their experience of this hard time. The difficulty lies in long working hours, an unfavourable workplace atmosphere, and limitations on their nursery use. Couples adopted various strategies to cope with these difficulties; adjusting their work pattern, reducing housework, calling on help from relatives, and so on. The childcare leave and childcare-break system are mostly regarded as helpful, but some pointed out defects. Couples negotiated with each other, seeking better arrangement. These experiences brought about changes in their attitudes, especially with the greater priority they placed on family life. Some said that having children limited their work capacity in some respects though being with them is priceless. Some talked about the needs for a 'decent track' in which they are free from the penalties of being parents.

Keywords Work-family interface · Dual career couple · Family life-cycle · Decent track · Couple interview

5.1 The Work-Family Balance: Impossible in Theory

Aiming to realise a gender equal society in which both men and women work full-time and equally share in the housework, the Japanese government announced two measures in 2004: the first to reduce childcare work and the second to cut the

Y. Senda, *Childbearing and Careers of Japanese Women Born in the 1960s*, Population Studies of Japan, DOI 10.1007/978-4-431-55066-2_5

hours of employed labour down to 1800 per year.[1] However, according to a simulation based on time-use data, the situation in which both men and women work full-time and equally share in housework will not be met even if the effects of these two measures are fully realized (Tanaka 2003). Even if work hours and childcare hours are reduced in accordance with the policy, there is no other way for a couple to juggle work and family unless they make arrangements for either the wife or husband to considerably reduce their work hours and increase time for childcare and housework.

The above situation is even more necessary in the current situation. While their child requires care, either the wife or husband must leave their job to devote themselves to housework and childcare, or work part-time in order to perform most of the housework and childcare.

However, there are actually cases, albeit a small number, in which both the wife and husband work full-time while raising children. They practice what theory implies is impossible. How do they live their lives?

Here, these questions will be approached by conducting interview surveys among dual-income couples who work full-time while raising children, focusing on the life stage that present extreme difficulties in the work-family issue.

5.2 The Work-Family Interface

5.2.1 The Couple as Unit of Analysis

Schein (1978: 60) used a diagram to illustrate the work-family interface model for dual-career couples. He commented that the work-family interface for dual-career couples is dynamic, rather than static. Therefore, in order to uncover the reality of the work-family interface for dual-career couples, it is necessary to consider the wife and husband together as a unit of analysis.

Although the necessity of couple-based analysis was already pointed out as early as the 1970s, little research has been conducted since then. Kato (2010) analysed data on wife-husband pairs to see what effect one member's experience

[1]The Labour Policy Council of the Ministry of Health, Labour and Welfare reviewed the current Act on Temporary Measures Concerning the Promotion of Reduced Working Hours—which aims to uniformly reduce employed labour hours down to 1800 per year—and submitted a recommendation on December 17, 2004 stating that the work hours should be set based on 'considerations for individual's health and life'. The Ministry of Health, Labour and Welfare plans to revise the law based on recommendations, and lay out a new set of guidelines—issue-specific measures such as utilising various systems to encourage people working long hours to take paid vacations, or measures to delay the start of work on Mondays and the days after holidays so that employees who have to relocate away from their family for work can spend enough time with their family, and so on—that can be used as references.

of a work-family conflict had on the other. It showed that a wife's family → work conflict (a conflict due to the family role putting pressure on her achievements at work) and a husband's family → work conflict affected each other. It seemed that the wife's and husband's conflicts each affected the other because each communicates the state of their own family → work conflict to the other. The study confirmed that, as a method for dual-career couples to reduce work-family conflicts, there are measures to 'coordinate roles between wife and husband', 'reduce family roles', and 'enhance family roles' within the family domain. It was also hypothesised that there are measures to 'coordinate job responsibilities within the workplace', 'reduce job responsibilities', and 'enhance job responsibilities' in the work domain as well. The study pointed out that 'for an individual who is juggling work and family, it might be easier to execute the measures in the family domain' (Kato 2010: 149).

5.2.2 Conflict/Enrichment

The work-family interface has been studied since the 1950s. For many years, investigations have especially focused on the circumstances of work-family conflicts that were brought on by strain (Barnett 1996). For example, research on the work-family interface has substantially grown in industrial-organizational psychology and in organizational behaviour since the 1980s (Greenhaus 2008), where it focuses on how a negative mood in one sphere affects the other sphere and vice versa, resulting in negative 'spillover' or 'crossover' (Williams and Alliger 1994). The perspective that the work-family interface can also result in synergies has gradually arisen since the 2000s. For example, Voydanoff (2002) investigated role balance and role enhancement, while De Klerk et al. (2012) focused on work-family enhancement, positive work-family spill over, work-family facilitation, and work-family enrichment.

5.2.3 Interaction with Life Stages, Family Stages, and Career Stages

'Life stages' is part of the concept of the life–span in developmental psychology. Super (1980) proposed the life-career rainbow model of one's life as a developmental process consisting of six stages distinguished by age, and features every stage through the use of six roles that he defined as being linked to each other. His work suggests that the roles of worker and homemaker are both major roles, especially in one's early 30s, and that the importance of each overlaps, to some extent, with the other.

'Family stages'[2] is a concept that stemmed from 'life stages'. Duvall and Miller (1985) and Bigner (1994) put 'Married Couples without children/Newly Established Couple stage' before the 'Childbearing Family stage'. Family stages have an influence on the coping strategies taken to decrease the work family conflict (Schnittger and Bird 1990).

'Career stages' are based on the concept of a 'career cycle', proposed by Schein (1978). It consists of nine stages that cover the period from one's childhood to retirement. Here, the term 'career stages' will denote those nine stages according to the custom in industrial organization psychology, although Schein himself did not use the term.

Along with the rising attention given to the work-family interface, researchers have begun to investigate how differences among life stages, family stages, and career stages have influenced the work-family interface; the basic proposition is that life stages and family stages partly determine career development, and that different life and family stages bring out different experiences in the work-family interface. Research such as that of Erikson et al. (2010) and Demerouti et al. (2012) agreed that the relationship between work-role demands and work-family conflict is at its greatest in early adulthood and in the transition to the parenthood stage. An individual has to decrease work-family conflicts to a decent level in order to adapt herself or himself to a new life, family, or career stage.

5.2.4 The Impact of Childrearing

The birth of a child brings a significant change to married couples. Parents play a large role during the child's infancy, since raising a child is particularly demanding during that time. At the same time, working parents also have to play the role of a mid-level employee at the workplace. Therefore, it is important, and yet difficult, to balance these roles (Fukumaru 2000). As they transition from the family-life stage of being a 'childless couple' to that of a 'couple with a child', the couple must create new behavioural patterns based on their redefined roles (Trost 1974).[3]

---

[2]There is also an idea suggesting that not only children, but also their parents, develop in childrearing. Galinsky (1987) conducted an interview survey of 228 parents and arrived at the six-stage model of parenthood. The six stages are 'Image-Making Stage' (during pregnancy), 'Nurturing Stage' (from childbirth to the child's second year), and so on.

[3]Recently, the concept of 'transition cycle' (Nicholson 1987) was introduced to describe women's career development and to describe the manner in which one adjusted to new dimensions, such as marriage and childbirth (Kanai 2010).

5.2.5 The Purpose of This Study

In this chapter, we investigate the work-family interface of dual-income couples, mainly in their 30s, who have a baby. In their 30s, the demands derived from their family stage (as they begin to have a child) and their career stage (where they begin to receive promotions) are both larger and in greater competition with each other than before. We focus on that period of time between when one of the parents takes childcare leave and when they return to work, a time during which the arrangement of work and family between couples is crucial. We can see how they go through their parenthood stages. We can stand on both sides of the interactions between wives and husbands and compare their statements on the same situation or event, and so on, when needed.

5.3 The Survey

I conducted a series of interviews on balancing work and childcare among ten dual-career couples with children residing in the Tokyo metropolitan area (Senda 2006). The attributes of the surveyed couples are shown in Table 5.1. At least one spouse from each of the surveyed couples took a childcare leave. While the combinations of the couple's employer types and job categories widely vary, everyone is a white-collar worker. The combinations of employer types and job categories among subject couples are (described in the order of wife's sector, wife's position; husband's sector, husband's position): (1) foundation, clerical; private company, research, (2) private company, clerical; independent administrative agency, research, (3) private company, semi-*sogo-shoku*; private company, *sogo-shoku*, (4) private company, professional; private company, professional, (5) private company, technical; private company, technical, (6) private company, *ippan-shoku*; private company, sales, (7) local government, professional; local government, clerical, (8) private company, research; private company, *sogo-shoku*, (9) private company, professional/managerial; private company, sales/managerial, and (10) school, professional; private company, technical.

There were 9 survey subjects born in the 1960s and 11 subjects born in the early 1970s; therefore, there were more individuals born in the 1970s in the survey sample. Looking at the subjects as pairs, at least one of them in 6 of those 10 couples was born in the 1960s. Although it is difficult to judge, it can be said with some certainty that the tendencies of the 1960s cohort are reflected, to some extent, in the study results.

The snowball sampling method was used to sample the survey subjects. Both wives and husbands were included in the survey. They were separately interviewed first during the time at which one of them was on childcare leave, and a second time 8–11 months after the individual returned to work. The interview was conducted twice per subject, for a total of 40 interviews.

Table 5.1 Attributes of survey subjects

Couple ID	(1)		(2)		(3)		(4)		(5)	
Subject ID	<1>	<2>	<3>	<4>	<5>	<6>	<7>	<8>	<9>	<10>
Place of work	Foundation	Private company	Private company	Independent administrative agency	Private company	Private company	Private company	Private company	Private company	Private company
Job category	Clerical	Research	Clerical	Research	Semi-sogo-shoku	Sogo-shoku	Professional	Professional	Technical	Technical
The year of marriage/cohabitation	2001		1999		1996		2001		1996	
Number of children	1		1		1		1		2	
Educational background	College	Graduate school	College	Graduate school	College	College	College	College	Graduate school	Graduate school
The year getting employment	1987	1992	1993	1997	1993	1993	1993	1994	1995	1986
The year of birth	1968	1968	1970	1969	1970	1970	1970	1969	1970	1963

(continued)

Table 5.1 (continued)

Couple ID	(6)		(7)		(8)		(9)		(10)	
Subject ID	<11>	<12>	<13>	<14>	<15>	<16>	<17>	<18>	<19>	<20>
Place of work	Private company	Private company	Local goverment	Local government	Private company	Private company	Private company	Private company	School	Private company
Job category	*Ippan-shoku*	Sales	Professional	Clerical	Research	Sogo-shoku	Professional/ managerial	Sales/ managerial	Professional	Technical
The year of marriage/ cohabitation	1997		2000		2001		1995		1993	
Number of children	2		2		1		2		3	
Educational background	College	Vocational school	Graduate school	College	Graduate school	College	College	College	College	Graduate school
The year getting employment	1993	1992	1998	1995	1998	1996	1990	1990	1989	1990
The year of birth	1970	1971	1973	1970	1973	1973	1967	1967	1966	1960s

The interviews were conducted in a semi-structured way. I prepared the main questions to cover matters such as occupational career, family career, history, and the length of childcare leave taken, as well as how work and family had been/are balanced, feelings toward balancing work and family, sharing housework and childcare with the spouse, the future outlook for work and family, and the desired measures for supporting their work-family balance.

5.4 Results

In what follows, comments will be quoted from the survey subjects. Each speaker is identified by their survey subject ID (<1> through <20>), which is listed in Table 5.1. An odd number indicates that the comment was made by a woman, and an even number indicates that the comment was made by a man. The couple is identified by their subject couple ID ((1) through (10)), also listed in Table 5.1.

5.4.1 The 'Both on Work with no Children Stage'

5.4.1.1 On the Intention to Continue Employment

There was no case in which the husband thought about quitting his job after his marriage. As for wives, some were certain that they would continue working for a long time, while others thought that they would try to continue working for the time being.

> Because those who work even after getting married began increasing around the time I started working for this company, it made me hope I could continue working at least until I bear a child. I thought I would continue working for the time being because I could quit any time. <11>

> I made it clear to him in advance by saying 'I will continue working no matter what. If you don't like it, I cannot marry you'. I said the same thing to his parents as well. I cannot quit halfway because I finally realised my dream. <19>

There was no case in which the wife wanted her husband to quit working upon marriage. There were, however, cases in which the husband wanted his wife to quit working upon their marriage.

> At first, I wondered why my wife would want to keep working after marriage, when women were allowed to quit the company upon marriage. <10>

> My husband was completely against the idea of me working after we got married because he grew up in a home where his mother was a full-time housewife. His younger sister is also a full-time housewife. We discussed it endlessly. We also argued about many other issues in preparation for marriage. My husband realised through discussions that I will not compromise. I think he ultimately thought 'Let me allow her to work for now and see how it goes'. <9>

5.4.1.2 On the Lifestyles Before Having Children

There were many cases in which the wife and husband each had their own lifestyle until they had a child.

> I never thought my life would change just because I got married. I thought each of us could work and have fun doing whatever we wanted. You don't have to change each other's life just because you got married. I thought it was good enough that we both go home to the same place. <3>

5.4.1.3 On the Timing of When to Have a Child

In many cases, the wife's opinion prevailed in terms of when she would bear a child. The remarks for this included: (1) 'I wanted to have a baby early. There is an age limit at which you can bear a child' on the wife's side; (2) 'I didn't want to have a baby right after getting married. But she did. So, we had a baby soon after we were married' on the husband' side.

The husbands prioritised their wives' opinions out of the consideration that women would leave their jobs for childbirth.

> Balancing work and childcare must be much harder for my wife. She has to take time off from work for a certain period and then transfer to another department after taking time off. When you repeat this two-to-three times, your career is ruined. Men don't sacrifice anything. <4>

However, it was not always the case that couples could conceive a child right after deciding they wanted a child. More than one couple indicated that they could not easily conceive or that they underwent fertility treatment. There was also a case in which the couple did not become pregnant while the work was demanding, even though they were engaged in acts designed to make them pregnant, but became pregnant once their workload was reduced. This process suggests that this is a factor for fecundity.

> When I had finally finished a demanding 6-year project, they immediately assigned me another 6-year project. I thought I could never bear a child as long as I'm on such a hard project. Although I put up with it for one year, I petitioned directly to my boss to take me off the project. Soon after that, I got pregnant. I'm the kind of person who doesn't get pregnant easily. Although we tried to get pregnant while I was on the project, I didn't get pregnant. I think it's because I was so stressed out. <19>

5.4.2 The 'Expecting Stage'

5.4.2.1 On the Intention for Continued Employment

There was no case in which both the wife and husband thought about quitting their jobs upon pregnancy. No subject wished that their spouse would quit working, either. Note that there were some wives who thought 'I would continue working if certain conditions are met' rather than 'I will definitely continue working'.

Quite a few people asked me 'You are going to keep your job even when you have a baby, aren't you?' and it puzzled me why people would ask such an obvious thing. I was actually amazed just how many people assumed a woman quits her job when she has a baby. <7>

When I found out that I was pregnant, I decided to go ahead and take maternity leave and one-year childcare leave. I decided to think about what I'll do after that when the time came. <13>

Once couples find out they are pregnant, they begin thinking that some kind of work arrangement is needed in order for both of them to continue working full-time after their child is born. The remarks for this included: (1) 'I mentally prepared myself to gradually reduce my workload so that both of us can continue working, if that's possible'; (2) 'Since both of us were working until late at night, I thought one of us had to change the way of working.'

5.4.2.2 On the Reactions at the Workplace

On the Supervisors' Reactions to Childcare Leave Requests

In cases where a request for leave was made in a workplace in which there were enough other workers who had already taken childcare leave, requests for leave went smoothly.

Everyone at the workplace simply assumed that I would take a one-year leave and come back. So, when I informed my boss I was pregnant, it was like, 'Sure, you'll be back in one year then'. <11>

In a case where the study subject made the first request in the workplace, the reaction was positive, but with some bewilderment.

Although it didn't go smoothly because I was the first one to take childcare leave in my workplace, they processed my request kindly. When I informed my boss I was pregnant, he asked me what I wanted to do with my job. I said 'I would like to take childcare leave'. My boss didn't say he approved or disapproved. He just asked me what he should do with the work that I was handling. <1>

When I said I was pregnant, my boss became gloomy like it was a funeral. I think he was at a loss as to what to do because I was single-handedly managing the staff and now I was going to be away all of sudden. It took a long time before my boss said 'Congratulations on your pregnancy'. After that, while I told him 'I'm planning to continue working', I was thinking it was depressing like we were at someone's wake. <3>

Although my section chief didn't bat an eye when I informed him I was pregnant, I heard later that he was completely taken aback. Those people just don't think there is a possibility for pregnancy, which in turn, interferes with the work. I bet they never imagined that I might become unavailable as manpower, given that my department at the time did not have female staff placement until recently. That said, because the department head is a very liberal person, he accepted it indifferently by saying 'It happens. So don't make her work too hard'. <7>

On the Transfer of Work in Preparation for Childcare Leave

The work a subject was handling when she/he requested leave was handed over to another person at various points in time by various methods after the pregnancy was reported and just before her maternity leave or his childcare leave. Of the 11 individuals who took childcare leave, there were four cases in which the individual allocated or handed her/his work to colleagues before going on leave and two cases in which a successor was automatically placed because the individual took leave during a routine personnel rotation at the company. There were five cases in which substitute personnel were assigned to the individual on childcare leave. Of those, four were temporary employees.

At workplaces where nobody had ever taken childcare leave before, the supervisor would sometimes ask the individual how her work should be transferred to others. In these cases, she would make decisions on her own as to how her work should be allocated, and ask her colleagues to take over her work before going on the maternity leave.

> My boss asked me how the work should be handed over to others and what kind of person should be hired as a substitute. He asked me when and how he should have substitute personnel ready. <1>

There were two cases in which the supervisor reduced the individual's work immediately after she informed them of her pregnancy. It made these individuals highly satisfied, because they felt they received direct support from the workplace, and the workflow became smooth because the supervisor gave clear instructions to the other staff members concerning what tasks could or could not be assigned to the pregnant individual, ultimately reducing the risk on the body of the expectant mother by reducing her workload from early on in her pregnancy.

> When I informed my boss about my pregnancy, she immediately looked up things such as tasks that pregnant women are exempted from and divided what work I could and could not continue to handle. It was great because clear instructions like that made people around me aware what tasks they can assign to me. My boss is the kind of person who would state out loud that pregnancy isn't a disease. Her considerate acts helped me, as well as the people around me. <13>

> When I informed my boss about my pregnancy, he knew how hard things are during pregnancy and cut my work as much as possible because being busy is not good. He also eliminated work that requires travel. My work was cut in half after I told him about my pregnancy. At first, I myself honestly thought he didn't need to cut so much of my work, but looking back, it was about right. After all, you cannot work until late at night while pregnant. Since my work was cut in half, I was able to leave the office on time most of the time. In order to commute by train that is not crowded, I changed my schedule to go into the office at 10:30 a.m. And leave at 7:00 p.m. <15>

5.4.2.3 On the Physical Conditions During Pregnancy

More than half of individuals who have had a baby mentioned that they experienced some issues at work stemming from their physical condition during pregnancy. There were many cases in which concerns that the development of foetus might be affected, albeit temporarily, arose.

> I began using paid time off to rest because the growth of my child declined just prior to starting the maternity leave. I was working normally until then. I wasn't hospitalised; I rested at home. I think I was probably tired because it was a busy season at work. <1>

> I used to feel ill about once a month during my latter pregnancy period. I would feel a tightening of the stomach by the second half of the week and it felt like the baby was coming down when I was standing. Once, my stomach was hurting so much that I went home by taxi. I took time off if I didn't feel well when I got up in the morning. During the month prior to starting my maternity leave, I made sure to request a day off every week in advance, regardless of how I was doing. It was hard to go up and down the stairs. I didn't want to be threatened by premature delivery after safely reaching latter pregnancy period. <5>

> I was completely exhausted towards the end because the latter period of my pregnancy and the office relocation came at the same time. I also worked overtime often. It was hard after the relocation because I also had to transition my work to others. I took a paid day off once when I had summer heat fatigue after wrapping up my work. I was resting at home all day for about half a month after I went on my maternity leave. When I went to the hospital, they gave me a slip for pregnancy-induced hypertension and I thought to myself 'this isn't good'. <11>

> I worked while taking Utemerin, a drug that suppresses preterm labour. Since my stomach was pretty heavy, I thought I might go into premature labour. <17>

Subjects who lived in a metropolitan area faced many issues related to commuting while pregnant, such as the morning rush hour and long commutes.

> Commuting to work while being pregnant was hard because the train was crowded. It was so hard that I once shouted in spite of myself 'Excuse me, don't push me, you are pressing my stomach!' because my stomach almost got squeezed. Everyone is desperate to get on the train, you know. So I tried to go as early as possible. I researched which train is less crowded and where in the train is less crowded. <17>

> I used to commute to work insanely early in the morning in order to get a seat in the train. I would leave home around 6:30, because no one would give up a seat for me just because I'm pregnant. <19>

5.4.2.4 Childcare Leave

The State of Childcare Leave Utilisation

Of the ten couples surveyed, nine used only the wife's childcare leave while the remaining couple used both the wife's and husband's childcare leave. Five out of the ten couples had one child, and the wives took only one childcare leave. Three couples had two children and the wives took childcare leave once per child, a total of two times. Since in one couple, both the wife and husband used childcare leave, they took childcare leave twice even though they only had one child. One couple had three children (including one set of twins). The wife took childcare leave once when they had the first child and once more for the twins, a total of two times. Therefore, a cumulative total of 15 individuals in 10 couples took childcare leave. Only one of them was male.

Why Do Only Wives Take Childcare Leave?

In Japan, the people who take childcare leave are predominantly women. According to statistics from 2012, the rate of childcare leave among employed workers who have children was 83.6 % for women and 1.89 % for men. The breakdown by gender for individuals who have taken childcare leave is 96.2 % women and 3.8 % men (*Basic Survey of Gender Equality in Employment Management 2012*).

Why is it that those who take childcare leave are all women? First, there were many cases in which the wife ended up taking childcare leave because both she and her husband found it hard to imagine the husband taking childcare leave.

> I never thought of taking childcare leave. The idea of a man taking childcare leave does not exist at my workplace. I myself cannot imagine a man taking childcare leave. <6>

> I never thought of asking my husband to take childcare leave, although I secretly wished he did when we had our second baby. I knew that his company had no understanding whatsoever for men to take childcare leave. I also knew that my husband didn't have that kind of idea at all. <7>

Second, as people climb the career ladder, they must continue to work hard. Most husbands hesitated to take childcare leave because they intended to be promoted, while most wives did not have any intention of being promoted. The reasons for this included: (1) 'I have no intention to advance to a management position. I'm prepared to have a break in my employment upon having a baby' on wife's perspective; (2) 'Taking childcare leave to create a break in occupational life feels like stepping down. That stops me from taking the plunge' on husband's perspective.

Third, from husbands' perspective, they did not need to take childcare leave because their wives put the husbands' career before their own. The reasons for this included: (1) 'My job is prioritized over my wife's job by her'; (2) 'When one of us must bear the burden, my wife always takes it for me'.

What Prompts Husbands to Take, or Consider Taking, Childcare Leave?

In what situations would husbands take, or consider taking, childcare leave? This study identified the following factors:

1. Critical situations that cannot be overcome by only one person

With Couple (4), the husband took childcare leave for five months after the wife took her childcare leave, until the child turned one. They made this choice due to an unexpected situation in which they could not enrol their child in a nursery before the wife had to return to work.

> I was shocked when we couldn't enrol our child in a licensed nursery (they meet the standards set by the government) because I had taken it for granted. I mean, we even relocated for that. We tried the next best thing, to enrol our child to an unlicensed nursery, but it didn't work out, either. It came down to either asking my wife to take another childcare leave or taking childcare leave myself. So I decided to take it myself. It took me a while to think it through, but I made all decisions in one sitting at one point. I made

> up my mind because I thought it was wrong to impose the responsibility onto my wife. I thought it is irresponsible to force her to take childcare leave and not to use my right to take childcare leave when I also had it. My wife handled all childcare while she was on the leave. I took no part in childcare. I vaguely wondered if I feel okay about not fulfilling any responsibility as a father. That was another reason that I took childcare leave. <8>

2. Role Models at the Workplace

Some husbands proactively considered taking childcare leave (even though they actually did not). A common factor among them was that they, and their colleagues, thought it might have a ripple effect to other male workers around them if they became the first men to take childcare leave.

> We tried to take six-month childcare leave each. That way, I would be the first male to take childcare leave in our municipality. My colleagues said 'Do it, do it'. I was very disappointed when I found out I couldn't take childcare leave due to the circumstances at my wife's workplace. It was frustrating. <14>

In the case of Subject <14>, he and his wife planned to each take a half-year of childcare leave. However, his wife's workplace did not accept that, giving the reason that substitute personnel should be contracted for a full one-year term.

3. Interest in Focusing on Childcare

There was one case in which a husband wanted to take childcare leave due to an interest in childcare itself, thinking that he would like a period of time to take care of his child on full-time basis.

> In my mind, there is also an idea that childcare is probably easier than work. I also think I would like to try caring the child full-time. <14>

Do Wives Want Husbands to Take Childcare Leave?

Upon childbirth, maintaining a dual income while the wife took childcare leave was part of an unspoken agreement that did not even need to be discussed by the couple. The reasons for this included: (1) they never thought of a man taking childcare leave; (2) when a man takes childcare leave, he might fall off the promotion fast track; (3) the wife does not feel she can leave childcare to her husband; and (4) the wife wants to take childcare leave herself since it is the perfect opportunity to take time off.

5.4.3 'On the Childcare Leave Stage'

5.4.3.1 On the Housework and Childcare During Childcare Leave

Among those who took childcare leave, there were some people who regarded, and performed, housework and childcare as their work while on childcare leave.

> Since I'm on childcare leave, I take care of all housework and childcare. I think I just have to accept it. <8>

However, conflicts over how to share housework and childcare arose between the partners when the partner who took childcare leave viewed childcare as their only responsibility. The woman taking childcare leave thought she was equal to the partner who remained working at the company, because she handled childcare as if it was her job as well. Therefore, she thought the housework should be shared between them. The husband, who was not on childcare leave, thought it was only natural that his partner handled both the housework and childcare because, while he was 'outside', his partner stayed at home. This disagreement caused a conflict over how the shared the housework.

> I'm annoyed when he says I'm supposed to make dinner because I'm home all day. It's true I'm home all day, but my job is to take care of our child. His work outside and my childcare at home are equal. So, I think he could make dinner half of the week. My husband's opinion is different. I'm currently on childcare leave, but there are various disputes over housework and childcare. <13>

> I think I'm handling as much housework and childcare as I can. I think I'm the one under a pretty tough condition needing to balance work, housework, and childcare. That said, whether my wife is satisfied is a completely different story. She gets mad that my share is small. I admit that the work I perform at home isn't enough. But to me, I'm doing as much as I can. I wish my wife understands that. <20>

There was an idea that it could not be helped if the partner could not share in the housework and childcare because he worked long hours at the office; not bringing family matters to work are customary when someone is under such a situation. The following quotes are from Couple (3):

> My view is that it's not my husband's fault but the company's fault that he doesn't do childcare. At my husband's company, unpaid overtime work is expected. That is the problem for childcare. I don't think it's normal to do so much overtime work. But if he gets lower evaluation and misses promotion for stopping working overtime, he won't feel fulfilment at work. So, I haven't expected him to help in childcare from the beginning. <5>

> My wife and I are both working after all and since we are living together, I know I can't escape from childcare work, nor do I want to escape from it. Coming home late from work is not good. I feel it's inhumane. I would like to live like a normal human being. My colleagues also say so. But, for some reason, I can't stop working overtime. <6>

5.4.3.2 On the Lifestyles of Those Who Did not Take Childcare Leave

Once a child is born, the importance of the family domain increases whether or not a parent takes childcare leave.

> Things changed dramatically after the baby was born. I stopped working through the night at the office. <4>

> I began trying to go home early after we had a baby. I tried not to volunteer for unnecessary work and asked others to handle what I can delegate. <10>

However, still, they work hours. There are cases in which the husband cannot involve himself in housework and childcare because he is exhausted from long hours at work.

> I'm thinking I have to help in childcare a bit, but I'm too tired to bring myself to do it. <6>

5.4.3.3 Life with Uncertain Future

With dual-career couples, there were many uncertain elements regarding their future outlooks for work as well as childcare. Either spouse could be rotated to another job or transferred to another location. There was no telling whether their child will become accustomed to going to the nursery. They never knew when they could get a task that could not be delegated, even though they needed to pick up their child at the nursery. They did not know when their parents—who were helping them care for the child—would begin requiring care giving themselves.

The strategy for dealing with these uncertainties in life was to take the stance that 'we can choose a different path at any time'. With this thinking, couples just needed to make the immediate choice that was suitable for their given situation. However, that did not eliminate their anxiety.

> I just can't really think about the future. I don't know if my child will get used to the nursery. I don't know what I'll do when my child gets sick. I don't know how we can take turns picking up our child at the nursery. I'm completely preoccupied thinking how we can manage this as a couple. It's so depressing. <8>

5.4.4 'Return to Both at Work Stage'

5.4.4.1 Daily Life: Not a Moment to Spare

Dual-career couples have to take care of housework and childcare before going to work and after coming home—and whenever they were at home—within a limited amount of time.

> I'm busy in the morning and evening. I'm always busy during the hours that I'm home. <13>

We will specifically look at how busy their schedules were in the morning.

> I experience an incredible level of busyness in the morning. <2>

> At first, my husband was helping the older child change clothes and I was helping the younger child change clothes in the morning. But before I knew it, I was the one helping both children change clothes. I try to wake them up, but they don't wake up easily. I have to dress the children like dressing dolls, while they are still half asleep and can't stand up straight. That was too difficult for my husband to do. He takes out the garbage in the morning. It seems taking out the garbage is the most he can do in the morning. <9>

As described, dual-career couples were busy in the morning. However, they were even more busy at night which was even worse because they have to put children to bed at an hour that is not only predetermined but also early. The average time between when a parent comes home and when they put their children to bed is three hours. They have to play with their children, prepare and eat dinner, give their children a bath, and tuck them into bed. Their busy schedule continues even after the children fall asleep, because they have to do housework.

> I go pick up my child at the nursery by 6:30 p.m. We come home at 7:00 p.m. We start dinner at 7:30 p.m. I do the dishes at 8:00 p.m. Then we take bath. My child goes to bed by 10:00 p.m. I wish I could put my child in bed by 9:00 p.m., but I can't. There are too many things to do after coming home and before tucking my child into bed. In order to begin preparing dinner at 7:00 p.m. and serve dinner at 7:30 p.m., I use pre-cooked food products so that I can just heat it up or boil it. <1>

> In the morning, I get to the office at 7:50 a.m. I work until 4:30 p.m. and go pick up my older child at the nursery at 5:20 p.m. I meet my mother at the nearest train station from the nursery to pick up my younger child whom my mother takes care of until then. When everything goes smoothly, we get home by 6:40 p.m. We have dinner at 7:00 p.m. We start taking bath at 7:45 p.m. I begin tucking my children into bed at 8:30 p.m. My older child goes to sleep by 9:00 p.m., but my younger child sometimes doesn't go to sleep until close to 10:00 p.m. Once my children are asleep, I get up and pack lunch for the next day for myself and my husband and make dinner for my husband. <9>

5.4.4.2 The 'Use Whatever Came to Hand' Method

Getting Over the Heavy Workload: The Work Sphere

1. **Using a Childcare-break System**

Employees can use a childcare-break system (a system with shorter work hours that allows childcare) if the employer offers it. The childcare-break system has been viewed as very effective for balancing work and family by its users. They perceived it as a system that not only directly supports childcare but also helps to spread the burden of housework and reduces the burden of commuting, for example. In addition, using the childcare-break system has the secondary effect of reducing the burden of commuting for parents who are pregnant with another child.

> My work hours are from 9:30 a.m. to 4:30 p.m. (full-time work hours are 9:00 a.m. to 5:00 p.m.). I use the childcare-break system. Initially, I was working from 9:30 a.m. to 4:00 p.m., which allowed me to get home a little after 5:00 p.m. but since it was difficult to carry out the work when the hours end at 4:00 p.m., I decided to extend the hours by just a little to 4:30 p.m. As for the morning, I have shortened my work hours by 30 minutes because there is a commuter rush in the morning and it also takes me a while to get ready to leave home. I think I am able to balance work and family because my child is in good health and my work hours are short. I would be walking on the wire if I were working full-time. It's probably not possible unless I have one more support system, such as a babysitter. <15>

> Because I was using the childcare-break system to shorten my work hours after having the first child and I didn't have to commute during the rush hours, commuting to work while being pregnant with my second child was easier. <19>

However, sometimes employees could not use the childcare-break system because of the atmosphere at their workplace.

> According to the company provisions, you can use the childcare-break system until your child turns six. But I'm not going to use it. I can't just say 'I'm leaving at five o'clock' and go home when everyone else is staying. I can't do it because my colleagues might stop regarding me as part of the team if I did that. <5>

<5> was using flexitime instead of the childcare-break system. However, another problem might occur alongside this practice (see Sect. 5.4.6.2).

Some of the survey subjects were working overtime even when they were using the childcare-break system. They did so to justify their use of the childcare-break system to colleagues who worked not only full-time but also overtime. When someone used the childcare-break system, their salary was reduced in accordance with their new work hours. However, they still worked longer than the specified hours.

> I am using the irregular and shorter work hour system. I'm the first management personnel who used the shorter work hour system. I work until 12:30 on Monday, Wednesday, and Friday and work full-time on Tuesday and Thursday. My total work hours are cut to 70%. But, I almost never actually leave the office at 12:30. I work until four o'clock most of the time. I end up working until around eight o'clock on Tuesday and Thursday.
>
> I work until four o'clock even though my hours end at 12:30 on the contract because it acts as a buffer to prevent my subordinates from complaining that I only work short hours even though I'm the manager with a higher pay. I don't get paid for overtime even when I work until four o'clock. Everyone else is doing two to three hours of overtime every day. If they think 'She's doing unpaid overtime work', it's unlikely that they will feel unfairness even if I go home early. That way, when the school has parents' day, for example, it is easier for me to say 'I'll leave the office at one o'clock today because I have to go to parents' day'. I mean, I'm on a contract to work only until 12:30 to begin with. <17>

As a manager who works shorter hours while everyone else works long hours, <17> devised a way of working that earned the support of her subordinates. However, her husband was dissatisfied with the way she worked because it increased his share of the childcare responsibilities.

> My wife wants to go to work on weekends because she works short hours. I don't really think it's a good thing. I don't like it. I say this because a couple should raise children together. We are both equally off on weekends. So we should equally divide childcare. And yet, I have to take care of the child by myself on weekends. That's not fair. That is my complaint. <18>

2. **The Changing their Ways of Working Pattern**

In the case of jobs that could be performed at the employee's own discretion, some individuals balanced childcare and work by changing their work patterns. However, the type of occupations that allow such independent work required long work hours to begin with.

It has become a routine, since the beginning of this year, for me to come home once in the evening to have dinner with the child, give him a bath, and tuck him in bed, and then go to work one more time. <4>

I'm a sales person who makes rounds outside. My job is to go see my corporate clients. My company requires me to always return to the office at the end of the day. But I changed the way I work so that I go directly to my clients from home and then directly go home from my clients. I used to visit one client per day, but I'm visiting two clients per day now. Once or twice per week, I go back to the office after visiting my clients. If it's not absolutely necessary, I won't go to the office. Regardless of whether going to the office every day or not, your job of who is to be assigned to you doesn't change when you are an outside sales person, you know. <12>

I can make time for childcare any time as long as my schedule is open. I was taking care of my child until noon today, too. My job allows me to use my discretion. <18>

3. **Devising Ways of Processing Jobs**

In order for both the wife and husband to be reinstated after childcare leave and continue working, it was essential for them to devise ways of adapting in the work domain. Ingenuity in the work domain was reflected in how one carried forward their work.

I can anticipate most things at work. I prepare for work ahead of time. I try to be prepared as much as possible so that I can take time off whenever I need for my child. <1>

It is very hard for both of us to be working when there is a child. So, I just try to complete all tasks while I can. I would steadily work ahead of schedule. But since administrative processes cannot be worked on ahead of schedule, there is a limit to what I can do. <8>

Reducing Housework: The Family Sphere

1. **Introducing Electrical Appliances**

Once couples found a need for reducing housework, their first step was to introduce automatic electrical appliances.

We automated housework. I bought appliances like a dishwasher and washing machine with dryer because my wife said 'Buy me appliances if you are not going to do housework'. If money can solve the housework problem, we solve it with money. In other words, we want to buy time with money. <16>

2. **Using Home-Delivery Services for Daily Necessities**

Utilizing home-delivery services could be also a good example of labour-saving techniques for housework.

I use pre-cooked foods from the co-op that I can just warm up or boil because I really want to be able to start fixing dinner at 7:00 p.m. and have it ready by 7:30 p.m. <1>

3. **Purchasing Professional Housekeeping Services**

In terms of using professional housekeeping services, there were aspects for which the opinion of the wife and husband differed. In these instances, the wife had positive views and the husband had negative views. The same was true for babysitters. It seemed that men felt resistance toward using money to buy housekeeping and childcare services from private companies and toward leaving housekeeping and childcare to complete strangers (see Sect. 5.4.5.2).

> We pay a professional cleaning service to come for all wet areas once every two weeks. It's been almost five years. It's expensive, but they clean the area really good. But that's not enough. I clean a little myself as well. <17>

> I was initially against hiring a professional to clean the house. My wife says she would rather spend time with children if she had the time to clean. But I thought she should quit working if that was the case. That said, outsourcing is very common in my industry. I thought about it and changed my mind that maybe it was okay to outsource cleaning as well. When I said 'I won't pay for that cost. We originally agreed that you take care of cleaning. Since you are the one outsourcing cleaning, you pay for it yourself. Do you agree?' She said, 'That's fine'. So I told her 'In that case, you go right ahead and outsource it'. I hate that we have to give the service provider the key to our house. I wish there was a guarantee that you can absolutely trust the service provider, but there is no such a thing. So, the first condition that I imposed was that they come when someone is home. My mother-in-law comes once a week to help with housework and childcare. So we have the cleaning company to come on those days. The terms that I set are for my wife to pay for the service and we have the service performed when her mother is there. <18>

4. **Preventing the Creation of Housework**

There was a case in which a couple reduced their housework by preventing it from being created.

> We don't have a dishwasher. We basically don't eat at home. So we have no dishes to wash. <8>

5. **Streamlining Housework**

Streamlining housework was extremely important for the double-income families with children. However, sometimes either the wife or husband could not fully and positively accept the streamlined housework if it felt like it was below their standards. We will use Couple (6) as an example:

> If I want to make curry now, it takes me six minutes before it's done. If I just throw some frozen mixed vegetables and ground meat in a pot, pour hot water from the thermos, and then add curry powder once it boils, it'll be ready in six minutes. It would be nice if I had 30 minutes to cook. If I had 30 minutes, I can make chopsuey in a wok and serve it over rice, for example. But I'd rather eat sooner than spend 30 minutes for cooking. <12>

> When my husband is cooking, sometimes I just want to say 'Your cooking is no good. Let me do it'. I shouldn't complain when he's cooking for us, but I wish he would cook something more decent. <11>

Couple (6) was in the stage of seeking new standards for their level of adequately streamlined housework. Couple (7) showed how they reached a point that was mutual acceptable (see Sect. 5.4.7.3).

5.4.4.3 The Trial-and-Error Method

The underlying factor that often required couples to rearrange how they shared their housework and childcare responsibilities, as well as their daily schedule, in a trial-and-error manner was the uncertainties surrounding the situation of their children. They could not tell what life patterns would work until they tried them, because the mood and health of their children varied by the situation.

> Since the beginning of this year, it has become my life pattern to come home once in the evening to have dinner with my family, give my child a bath, put him in bed at 9:00 p.m. and then go to work one more time. Earlier, our child used to go to bed at 11 p.m. When we changed our child's bedtime to 9:00 p.m. during the New Year holidays, his physical condition improved considerably. So, in order to keep putting him in bed at 9:00 p.m. after the New Year's holidays, I changed my life pattern. It makes it easier for me to work, too, when he is feeling well. <4>

> When my wife is alone with our children in the evening, she can't cook because she has to constantly deal with our younger child. Once clung to us, the younger one won't let us go. When my wife had just gone back to work from the childcare leave, I was getting home around nine. But when I got home at nine, groceries were still on the table and dinner wasn't prepared. The hungry children were waiting for dinner at nine o'clock. My wife was panicking trying to deal with the younger child. I thought this was not going to work. So, I began buying and stocking up processed foods such as rice balls and sandwiches which can be eaten easily. But my wife says she cannot even eat dinner by herself because she has her hands full taking care of the younger child. Since there was no other choice, I decided to come home early in the evening to cook dinner. You see, I can cook dinner quicker than my wife. My wife looks after the children while I cook. Then, we eat dinner.

> At the beginning, my wife had said 'Since I have energy left, I can make dinner, feed our children, and put them into bed all by myself'. But when she actually tried, it wasn't possible. When my wife told me 'I just can't. I'm reaching a breaking point', I thought I put her under pressure. So I decided I would also come home early in order to fix dinner. <12>

5.4.4.4 Tightrope Walking: When Children Become Sick

Sometimes the children suddenly become ill. When the nursery notices a sick child, they order the parents to immediately come pick up the child. In these instances, first one of the parents will try to pick up the child. However, it was difficult for the dual-career couples to always handle sudden, urgent matters, such as a child's illness, by themselves. Sometimes it was difficult for both the wife and husband to take time off from work. When that happens, these couples often relied on their parents. If their parents live close enough to come over in about three hours after being contacted, then the couples would rely on them in case of an emergency.

> When I absolutely have to do the work, I ask my husband to go pick up the child. When neither my husband nor I can take time off, we ask my mother. But we've asked my mother only once. Either my husband or I make arrangements at work and go to pick the child. <1>

> We can tell our child's physical condition the day before. When he seems to be getting sick, we ask my mother-in-law 'We are sorry, but do you think you can look after our child tomorrow afternoon?' I take the morning off to look after the child. I then go to work at 1:30 p.m. because my mother-in-law would come at 1:00 p.m. <5>

> When our child is sick, one of us takes time off from work to look after him. But, sometimes neither of us can take time off from work. When that happens, we call my parents and ask they could come and look after our child. My mother can get to our house in about three hours after we call. My wife can manage if it's only for three hours until my mother gets here. <8>

> When both my wife and I absolutely cannot take time off from work, we take our child to my parents' house and ask them to take care of him. My parents keep him for several days until he fully recovers. <14>

In terms of taking time off or leaving work early without advance notice due to their child's sickness, the interviewees thought that the understanding of their colleagues was important and that such leave depended on their boss's discretion.

> My former boss once gave me a warning about leaving work early. I think it was because he personally didn't like women with children to work. I think my current boss has an understanding for leaving work early and taking time off unexpectedly due to child's sudden illness. He has never said anything to me. <1>

> Because I've taken childcare leave, my standing as 'a person who is caring for a child' is already established within the company. So when I say 'I need to leave the office for an hour because my child has a fever', everyone sort of accept it like 'Oh well, I suppose he has no choice'. <8>

> The benefit of announcing at my workplace that my wife returned to work is that I can go home early when something happens. They let me go home when I say 'I'm sorry, my child has fallen ill with a fever of 39 degrees Celsius'. <12>

> My boss also has a child. When his child gets sick, he would say to me 'I'm sorry, I'm going to work from home today. If you need me, call me on my mobile phone'. As fellow individuals who work while raising a child, we are used to each other's ways. So, when he takes time off suddenly, I cover for him. Because of this, I can now sort of use my time as I wish, which is good. But, if I were to work for someone else, the way I work would probably change. When that happens, I won't be able to care for my child as I do now. <18>

5.4.5 Utilising Childcare Resources After Returning to Work

5.4.5.1 Choice of Residence

Those dual-career couples who work in the Tokyo metropolitan area have also thought out about where to live in order to balance their work and family lives. It was essential that they be smart when choosing where to live, by using criteria such as proximity to at least one of their workplaces, the convenience of at least one of their work commutes, and availability of extensive, local childcare services.

The childcare resources they used after returning from childcare leave were either nurseries or parents. If the wife had the clear intention that, upon marriage, she would continue to work after having children, then the couple considered the wife's accessibility to work and the available childcare resources, and chose their residence accordingly. There were many cases in which the couple relocated after pregnancy. While the need for a larger space for the child was one of the reasons for their relocation, the most important factor in choosing the location of the residence was the accessibility of childcare resources.

Factors such as whether the house was located close to their parents' house, if the community offered excellent childcare services, and the accessibility of the wife's workplace were particularly important when deciding where to live. The ease of the wife's commute is more often prioritised over that of the husband's because couples often planned for the wife to arrange her work hours in order to assume the responsibility of picking the child up from the nursery.

> We chose where to live by prioritising the ease of commute for my wife because we basically have no choice but to rely on my wife to pick up our child at the nursery. I think I could take the child to the nursery school in the morning, but I'm just going to have to ask my wife to pick him up. Moreover, my wife would have to drag her body to commute while she's pregnant. We chose the house based on the criteria that it is conveniently located for my wife to commute. <4>

There was also a case in which the couple considered the ease of commute and the adequacy of childcare services in their community upon learning they were pregnant, and chose to relocate to rental housing in order to live in the area for a while before eventually purchasing a house in that area.

> We moved here because the area offered good childcare. It certainly is good. For example, being able to leave the child at the nursery until ten o'clock at night is very reassuring. So, we decided to live in this area while our child goes to the nursery. Since the rent is expensive in this area, it's better to buy a house if you plan to live for several years. Another reason for buying a house is that we heard that the quality of the public elementary school is also high. <7>

5.4.5.2 Public Services: Nurseries and Their Substitutes

The people and entities who took care of couples' children while their parents worked during the day were nurseries, grandparents, and babysitters. One couple handed their child over to the child's grandmother. Two couples used two childcare services, the nursery, and a babysitter. Seven couples took their children to a nursery. Nurseries were the most frequently used childcare service. Nursery facilities were perceived as supporting parents who had to balance work and family and were also recognised as providing good care for children; they were generally highly regarded, whether they were licenced or not.[4]

> I think the nursery (qualified by local government) is very responsible. I don't have much to complain about. They call me when something happens to my child. When my child is bitten by another, they tell me 'He got bitten. They were fighting over a toy', for example. Since there is more than one nursery-school teacher per every three children, it's more than sufficient. <5>

---

[4]Some local governments set an original standard that is almost equivalent to that of the national government, with some exceptions such as whether it includes school grounds, etc. Nurseries that meet the local government's standards are qualified by the local government. All of the subject couples left their children with nurseries that were either licensed by the national government or qualified by their local government.

Some individuals were highly satisfied with the licensed nursery facilities (those that met the standards set by the government) based on the fact that they have a resident nurse and that the staff are experienced in childcare and offer extensive support.

> Sometimes the nurse would call me at around 5:30 in the evening and say 'I just took a temperature of your child and it was high. Since she's in a good mood and the nursery hours will end soon, we'll keep her here. I just wanted to let you know that she's feverish'. It means I should come to pick her up sooner than later. <11>

However, a wall stood in the way of some parents' appreciation of the services offered by the nursery. First of all, the availability of nursery facilities is low. In fact, there were some cases in which the parent who took childcare leave delayed the return to work, or both the wife and husband took childcare leave, because no nursery was available.

> The nursery told us 'We cannot start taking your child until this day'. I wanted to return to work a little earlier, but I rescheduled to suit the nursery's convenience. <5>

Furthermore, many regarded the inflexibility of the nursery's hours for childcare as a problem. In most cases, considering the time necessary for commuting, parents who worked full-time could not pick up their children on time, even if they left the office on time, unless they use after-hours childcare. Moreover, nurseries could not extend their childcare hours on the same day that it was requested. After a parent returned from childcare leave, whether they were able to always finish working in time to pick up their child from the nursery day after day was a significant concern that took an emotional toll on the couple. Some of the parents frequently contacted each other every day to ensure that whoever was available sooner could pick up their child from the nursery. There were days when both parents were busy at work, but nevertheless had to pick up their child. They contacted each other numerous times, making a decision at the last moment every time. It was as if they were walking the wire.

> I wish the hours of the nursery ended one hour later. I know there are other parents who come home late like us. I wish they took that into consideration and extended the childcare hours. <12>

The fact they have to make sure to pick up their children at the nursery at the same time every day put pressure on the parents.

> It would be nice if the nursery had more flexible hours. That way, the parents can work without worrying about the time. <14>

Another problem is that nursery facilities do not accept children who are sick. Parents had to pick up their children right away when they become sick at the nursery. The number of nursery facilities for sick children is limited, and they are not always in a convenient location. On the other hand, the reality at the workplace is that employees cannot take time off to care for their children, even when they are sick.

> When my child got sick, I just could not take time off. Because I'm the only one who can operate this machinery, the work won't get completed at the company if I wasn't there. Sometimes I asked my wife to take a day off. We have also asked her parents to keep our child for one to two weeks. We do have a ward nursery facility for sick children. But we never use it because it is far away. It is located really far away. <12>

The use of babysitters was also observed once the child became old enough. Two couples had already hired a babysitter at the time of the interviews. While women felt no resistance to hiring a babysitter, some of the men felt uncomfortable.

> I think we can get a babysitter when something comes up. But it seems that my husband feels uncomfortable hiring a babysitter. He says things like 'Is it safe to have a stranger in the house?' and 'It's cruel to place the child in a babysitter's care'. He thinks his parents are better than a babysitter. So, if I say 'I'll ask for a babysitter', he would say 'Wait. Let me ask my mother if she'll look after the child'. I'm uneasy about relying only on his mother. I think it's necessary to have multiple options for childcare providers ready just in case. <7>

5.4.5.3 Private Services: Assistance from Relatives

Six out of ten couples received regular assistance from their relatives.

> Sometimes I get an urgent job right before going home. When that happens, it's difficult. In such a case, I might ask my sister, who lives nearby, to pick up my child. Once or twice a month, my sister would volunteer by saying 'Since I can go home early today, do you want me to go pick up your kid?' It helps me a lot. <1>

> My mother-in-law comes to the house twice a week. She's working, too, but she gets off work at three o'clock. She comes around after that. She would go pick up my child at the nursery and cook dinner for us. Balancing work and childcare would be very difficult without her support. <5>

5.4.6 Bi-Directional Interference Between Work and Family

5.4.6.1 Family → Work Enrichment/Conflict

Work and childcare do not always conflict with each other. Sometimes they generated synergies:

> When I look at the growth of my child, my intellectual curiosity is stimulated quite a lot. Also, because children can be a common subject to talk about, it became easier to talk to people in older generations. <4>

However, many couples commented that, although the fulfilment they feel from having children is priceless, having children does have a negative effect on their work, because they have to put time and effort into their family. More specifically, the following examples of conflicts were mentioned: 'salary is reduced when taking childcare-break', 'the workplace does not understand that childcare imposes constraints on work hours', 'work is interrupted by childcare and housework', and 'because work hours are limited due to childcare even though the job mandates long work hours, it might negatively affect one's career development'.

> I reduced my workload in order to care of my child. I used to take on extra work after finishing my main work, but I stopped doing that, though that helped me when I worked on my next job. Now, I don't perform any work beyond what I'm required to do. It will probably come back to haunt me later. But there's nothing that I can do. <4>

> Dropping everything at work to come home, picking up the child, giving the child bath, tucking the child into bed, waiting until the child falls sleep, and then getting up again to return to work is a quite exhausting process. It interrupts your rhythm, which is hard, and it is physically demanding. There is a big gap when you have to think about the interpretation of the Constitution and the way that Japan should be after reading the children's book 'Guri and Gura'. <7>

> If I didn't have a child, I could have worked more. Aside from the question of whether that is good or bad, I probably could have devoted myself more to work had I married a full-time housewife. Many colleagues at my workplace hang out together at night for a drink. But I have to decline their invitation at night. I do feel unhappy about that. But I adore my child. When I think about the happy time that I spend with my child, the satisfaction that I get by spending time with my child is much larger than the dissatisfaction about declining to have a drink. I think I know the joy of spending time with my child because I had taken childcare leave. <8>

> I've been working shorter hours since we had a child. I used to go to the office at 6:00 or 7:00 a.m. and worked until around 11:00 p.m. or 12:00 midnight. I went to the office on most Saturdays and Sundays as well. Now that I have to drop off my child at the nursery, I can't go to the office as early in the morning as before. The earliest that I can start working is 9:00 a.m. I still work until late as before. But now that I have a child, I can't go to work on both Saturday and Sunday. I used to be ahead of others but now I'm trying to catch up to others. That part is tough for me. <16>

> I'm sure my colleagues would understand if I make a request by saying 'I'd like to go home early in order to care my child'. But it's unlikely that my colleagues will anticipate my need and say 'Why don't you go home early?' Until you become a parent, you cannot understand how hard it is. So, my colleagues are probably thinking that we are somehow managing even though my wife and I both work and I'm working overtime. <20>

In one case, the husband was worried about his wife's career development as well as her way of making arrangements for work. In particular, when both the wife and husband had highly specialised jobs, there were issues as to the extent to which each of them should coordinate, and whether such coordination was balanced between the wife and husband.

> When someone who is put in charge of a project suddenly takes time off, the supervisor probably wonders whether it's really okay to leave the work to that person. And the person probably wouldn't be able to do a good job when she/he takes time off. My wife probably wouldn't get any important assignment because the supervisor cannot be sure that she wouldn't take time off suddenly. That would be disadvantageous in developing her career within the company. So, I wonder to some extent whether my wife's career is okay. But I don't talk about that with her because if she says 'Well then, why don't you take time off for our child instead of me?' I can't say 'I will'. <16>

5.4.6.2 Work → Family Enrichment/Conflict

One study subject remarked that continuing to work enabled them to interact with their children in a better way.

> Work allows me to continue being myself. I can also better interact with my children when I'm interacting with them for a short time. The only way for me to interact with my children is to go pick them up at the nursery after finishing my work and have conversation with them like 'What did you do today?' 'I played with XX. I did this'. I'm sure there are parents who want to be with their children all day. I can't do that. What I can do is to spend a short, quality time. When I pick them up, I first hug them tight. That's how I communicate with my children. That's my way of showing love to my children. <19>

It was not uncommon for a subject to voluntarily request to be transferred to a department where balancing work and family is easier.

> I went back to the original workplace after reinstatement. But, as expected, the work was hard. My child began going to the nursery in April, and there have been many instances where I receive a sudden phone call because my child runs a fever. If I had to continue working in the original workplace, it would not be possible to go pick up my child at the nursery. Balancing work and childcare was indeed difficult. Then, the company was planning the routine job rotation (regularly exchange personnel between two departments). So I volunteered myself and asked if I could go to the other department starting in August. Well, the discussion went well and they said 'In that case, you can transfer', so I transferred. I knew that the individuals on routine job rotation served a two-year term and the next opportunity was coming up in August. I had always been interested in the work in the other department and wanted to go there at least once. I was waiting for the opportunity to transfer through the routine job rotation. Since the work is slightly easier at the other department, going there for two years will also buy me some time in terms of childcare until my child becomes old enough. I thought that would also work out well. Now that I've transferred, the work at my current department offers slightly relaxed time schedule. Because of that, things are much easier now in terms of time. This job is better suited for childcare because you are allowed to manage your time. I mean, it lets me work at home at night after my child goes to sleep. <8>

The case of Subject <8> was a very suggestive example of an individual who had a highly specialised occupation making a choice that values both their work and childcare as much as possible. He utilised the company's existing human resource management system and transferred to a department where he could 'temporarily' engage in work that he 'had always been interested in' and that was 'suitable for childcare from the perspective of allowing him to manage his own time'.

However, in another case, utilizing the existing human resource management system to integrate work and family brought poor results, at least in the work sphere.

> I work full-time by using the flexitime system. I go to work 30 minutes early and leave work 30 minutes early. But the flexitime system isn't supposed to be used all the time. I'm not sure what my colleagues think of me using it all the time. It's possible that they don't see it favourably. But I'm using it because I made it clear that was what I was going to do. As for the work, there is no way that I can handle it within regular work hours. Since the time to pick up the child at the nursery is fixed and I can't work overtime, I take it with me to work at home.

> I think I'm putting burden on my colleagues by using flexitime and going home early. But they are at fault, too. There is someone who submits a form for outsourcing work at the last minute and demand 'I'm submitting it today, so place the order today'. This person

> always come at around 4:30 p.m. and I think, 'But I'm scheduled to leave the office at 4:45 p.m'. When that happens, I somehow manage to place the order in 15 minutes. When we identify a mistake after placing the order, I correct it if I'm still there. But I would work overtime only through 5:10 p.m. because I'm determined to get on the 5:15 p.m. train. Sometimes I just want to cry because I'm always running to the train station. <9>

Subject <9> has a highly specialised job with inflexible work hours, because her job requires a lot of negotiations with both parties in the company and business partners outside the company. In order to balance her work and family, she devised a way of working in which she uses the flexitime system to begin working early in the morning and go home early instead. She cannot work much overtime because she has to pick up her children. Being on flexitime, her scheduled time to leave the office was 4:45 p.m. Because she had to pick up her child at the nursery at a specific time, the most overtime that she could work was until 5:10 p.m. In other words, she could only work 25 min of overtime per day (To be exact, she came to the office an hour earlier than she was required and also worked at home with no pay).

Among individuals who had the same type of job as Subject <9>, no one was working in a manner that allowed them to do almost no overtime work, or to leave the office on time. Subject <9> was stressed that she had to work in a different way than the others around her. She considered childcare important; she chose her current manner of work in order to balance work and family. At the same time, she desired to be recognised for her work. However, the company did not recognise her way of working. For example, although Subject <9> objectively showed her level of skill by taking and passing a qualification test, she was not promoted even though everyone else who had passed the same test received a promotion.

> Gradually, I began feeling 'I understand that working shorter hours in order to care a child is treated unfavourably in terms of personnel evaluation. But if that's the case, I will not perform any work beyond this scope since you rate me poorly'. <9>

5.4.7 The Dynamism of the Work-Family Interface

5.4.7.1 Processes for Reallocating Housework and Childcare

In terms of rearranging how housework and childcare responsibilities are shared when the spouse who is on childcare leave returns to work, the individual work situations faced by both the wife and husband became important factors. In many cases, the work situation differs between wife and husband. Since the wife and husband compare the level of difficulties facing each of them in the workplace, those housework and childcare responsibilities that are easier to balance with work were allocated to the individual with the harder job, while the responsibilities that are more difficult to balance with work were allocated to the individual with the relatively easier job. For example, the responsibility of shuttling the child to and from the nursery facility was divided so that the individual who will more frequently need to work overtime would drop the child off at the nursery, while the other individual would pick the child up. Since it is difficult to coordinate when both wife and husband have highly specialised jobs, or jobs with inflexible hours, they end up making arrangements that put a greater burden on one of them.

Transporting the Child to and from the Nursery

Couple (4) provides us with an example of the how to allocate childcare responsibilities after a spouse returns to work. They expected, and practiced, allocating responsibilities in terms of their job workloads. The wife also took into the consideration the fact that her husband pursued a greater responsibility for childcare compared to common husbands, going so far as to take childcare leave to make it possible for them both to continue working. She therefore thought it was her turn to take more responsibility in childcare; in this case, by taking the child to and from the nursery.

> I think it's difficult for him to leave the office by 8:30 at night every day. So, I'm thinking he can be the one to take our child to the nursery in the morning and I'll be the one to pick up the child at night. I think I'm going to have to keep taking more responsibilities for the time being, but since he did make a big decision to take childcare leave, I'm planning to give him room to breathe for a while. <7>

> I would like to return to the workplace I belonged to before I went on childcare leave, but it'll be difficult to balance with childcare because it is a department with very long work hours. I mean, I can't completely rely on my wife to shuttle the child to and from the nursery. I'm planning to take our child in the morning. Picking our child up is the problem. Since the nursery closes at 10:00 p.m., one of us must go pick up the child by then. I'm thinking about asking my wife to pick up the child at night for a while after I return to work. But I don't think I can ask her to do both every time. <8>

Regarding the process of establishing patterns for how to share the responsibilities of transporting their child to and from nursery after the husband returned to work, the couple each commented as follows:

> Since he was reinstated in the workplace that he belonged to before the childcare leave, dropping off and picking up the child at the nursery were really hard. He dropped off the child in the morning as often as he could, but he couldn't pick up the child at night at all. <7>

> After I returned to work, I tried to drop off the child in the morning as often as I could. I completely relied on her at night. <8>

Dropping off the Child at the Nursery or Housework

The manner in which a couple shared responsibilities was often established as their life pattern developed through trial-and-error. We will look at Couple (1) as an example.

> At the beginning, I was the one to take our child to the nursery. My husband was supposed to do housework instead, but he often forgot to take out the garbage and clean the house. So I told him I wanted him to take the child to the nursery so that I could do the housework.

> Initially after switching the responsibilities of taking the child to the nursery and doing the housework, I handled all the morning housework. Wake up the child, help the child

change the clothes, gather things to take to the nursery, prepare breakfast, pack our lunch, help the child eat the breakfast – I did all of them. So I was very busy in the morning. After a while, my husband began packing our lunch. Then, a while after that, he began preparing breakfast, although he was just putting bread on the table. Now that I don't have to pack lunch and make breakfast in the morning, my morning housework has become much easier. When you look at the entire housework, I think I'm handling more of it. But I'm happy about the fact I need to do less in the morning when it's chaotic. I've never pressured him into do more housework. <1>

I don't really remember how it happened, but I thought that things would be easier for my wife if I took our child to the nursery in the morning. So that's what I decided to do. As long as I'm doing something, I can talk back to my wife when she complains. I thought about what housework and childcare tasks to do and figured I should just do what I can do for now. It's not possible for me to go pick up our child at the nursery in the evening because I come home late from work. So I decided I'll take the child to the nursery in the morning.

As for sharing the housework and childcare responsibilities, we don't discuss it as a couple. Three of us live as a family. If I didn't do anything while my wife did housework, it would make me uncomfortable. I think I just need to take care of the housework and childcare tasks that I can. Since I like cooking, I'll fix meals. <2>

5.4.7.2 The Work-Life Balance Is a Work in Progress

One couple offers an example in which a sense of unfairness regarding how housework and childcare are shared transformed into a sense of fairness as the family stage evolved, and vice versa. Such transformations are endless. We will refer to the case of Couple (5):

I think the way we share the responsibilities of housework and childcare is becoming balanced recently. In my family, my wife decided how we should share housework and childcare responsibilities. Childcare is all handled by my wife. We divide housework between the two of us. I handle more housework than my wife since she takes care of the children. I didn't like this arrangement before because it looked like my wife had it easier. I think it is becoming balanced lately because as our first child is growing, my wife is doing a lot, such as getting various teaching materials to help him study and taking him to an English lesson. I'm beginning to see that my wife is actually spending considerable time for childcare. Based on what each of us can do, or how much time each of us has, I think the way housework and childcare are split is just right. When we got married, I wasn't sure if I could handle all the housework assigned to me. But, now that we have two children, the burden on the mother, who cares for them, has increased. So, based on the current state, I think I also have to do at least this much of housework. But, I can't handle any more than this. <10>

However, the husband in this case, who says 'I can't handle any more than this', felt that he is currently taking on the maximum amount of responsibilities that he can handle. The wife also felt that she had currently taken as many responsibilities as she could handle. In particular, the wife thought the housework and childcare burden that she took on was still heavier, even at present, and that the burden on her husband was lighter. She also felt that she was at the edge of her abilities.

He does take care of the housework that he was told to do, but I'm basically asking him to do housework that he doesn't want to do. Other people might look at this and think my husband is doing more housework than I am. But regardless of what people say, dealing with children is the hardest work in the world. I'm totally responsible for raising the children. My hands are full just for that. <9>

In response to this situation, Subject <10> suggested the possibility of readjusting the future work-family interface between him and his wife.

Recently, my wife has been saying this is physically too demanding. She just began saying it very recently, about one month ago. Before that, all she said to me was 'I'll keep working for the rest of my life'. It will be a really big deal if she quits her job. In terms of stability of life, it's better that both of us continue working. I've heard 'maintaining double income is a form of insurance'. That said, I can't force her. If she wants to quit working because she's tired, she should go ahead. My father was naturally the only one who worked in my family. My mother was a full-time housewife. I myself used to think it is normal for a wife to be a full-time housewife. The issue might be the state of mind or my wife might really be tired when she says she's tired. I do feel that perhaps I should help reducing her workload a little. <10>

5.4.7.3 Interaction Between Family Stages

To describe the interaction between work-family Interface and family stages, the case of Couple (7) will be quoted. While his wife was on childcare leave, the husband, Subject <14>, thought that the standard of housework imposed on him by his wife was too high for him to meet. However, he commented that the standard of housework that they each considered reasonable began to converge after his wife returned to work and they both began raising a child while working, because his housekeeping abilities improved and the standards his wife aspired to were lowered.

1. On the stage when the wife is on childcare leave:

As expected, balancing work, housework, and childcare is quite difficult. It's hard when you try to do all properly. You don't have to do everything perfectly, but my wife tries to do it properly anyway and also demands that I do it properly. It's difficult to do it at her level. I think it would be easier for her, too, if my wife was a kind of person who can cut corners, but she wouldn't do that. <14>

2. On the stage after the wife returns to work:

It seems that once both of us actually began working, my wife also realised that it is impossible to maintain the same housekeeping standard. Now, there is an unspoken understanding that ready-made side dishes are okay every once in a while. So, we buy them occasionally. Not so frequently though. The range of menus that I can cook is limited, such as curry, *niku-jaga* (a Japanese dish of meat and potato seasoned with soy sauce), and so forth. Since the cooking procedures are almost the same for curry and *niku-jaga*, I'm pretty good at it, too. Lately, it seems that my wife is gradually lowering her housekeeping standards. Sometimes she would say 'Why don't we get *shumai* and have it for dinner?' After actually trying it out herself, I think she realised it was hard to cook meals without relying on ready-made side dishes when you are working full-time. Since her required standard has come down, I haven't been annoyed by her complaints about how I do housework. <14>

5.4.7.4 Renewed Bonds Between Wife and Husband

Dual-career couples were re-establishing their marital relationships through coordinating their work and family in response to the changes in their family situation after having a child. This coordination, which begins during pregnancy, continues through the period during which one of the spouses takes childcare leave following the child's birth and continues through the first year after the spouse on childcare leave returns to work and the child begins to go to the nursery, during which their daily routine develops. In other words, the birth of a child makes the couple spend almost three years re-building their marital relationship by rearranging how they involve themselves in their family and their respective work.

In the course of the coordination process, explicit conflicts sometimes temporarily emerged between the wife and husband. Even in such cases, the couple built a new stable state that balanced work and family together by making further arrangements.

When they happened to face harsh situations, they somehow arranged a work-life balance, even though they often faced some complications that can always emerge among couples. Friction cannot always be avoided. Many couples renewed their relationship in a better way through addressing a conflict.

Regarding the feelings between the wife and husband at each stage—where in Stage 1 the wife becomes pregnant and takes childcare leave, in Stage 2 the wife returns to work and the husband takes childcare leave, in Stage 3 the husband returns to work, and in Stage 4 the husband transfers to another workplace about four months after returning to work—Couple (4) made the following comments, which we will review in order.

1. On the stage in which the wife becomes pregnant and takes childcare leave:

> I complained to him many times about the fact that I was always the one to do the housework while I was pregnant. I said 'Why do I have to be the one to do the laundry?' I happened to do the laundry only because I happened to be pregnant and not working until late at night, because I happened to be home earlier than him. I told him so many times that I really hate it when he expects me to do the laundry. I repeated to him many times 'Please don't take it for granted'.

> Even after the child was born, he still does not have a sense of ownership. No sense of ownership that he, too, is raising a child. At the time, he was leaving home at around 7:30 in the morning and coming home at around 2:00 in the morning. He usually slept until noon on his day off. I understand how hard the work is because I work in the same field. Still, I was of course unhappy. All those times, I thought 'Why can't he come home earlier?' I used to think it would make a difference even just by a little if he came home before midnight, for example. I wanted to tell him things like 'This is what happened today' or 'Our child accomplished this today'.

> At that time, I kept thinking how I'm overwhelmingly at a disadvantage; I got the short end of the stick by bearing a child, etc. Because he doesn't change the way he worked despite my repeated pleas, I was very unhappy, thinking 'Gosh, he really has no clue as a father'. I thought that perhaps it would be easier if I became a single mother rather than staying in this marriage so that at least I won't need to do his share of housework. <7>

> At my company, everyone in the same line of work as me works by sacrificing his family. All employees at my workplace are men. Since everyone is working that way, men are

expected to work by sacrificing family. I thought that was normal as well. To be honest, I felt I could not help it because of the nature of my work if I end up coming home late at night or could not do any housework or childcare. <8>

2. On the stage in which the wife returns to work and the husband takes childcare leave:

I began feeling less unhappy about my husband around the time when he became serious and said he would take childcare leave. I was supposed to return to work in September. About three months before that, around June, he began saying 'Shall I take childcare leave from September?' It turned out he was having a hard time bearing how I vented my dissatisfaction about him returning home late every weekend and not doing housework and childcare. I think he thought he had to do something. When he first said he'll take childcare leave, I was dubious. But because he began saying things like 'I consulted a senior colleague' and 'I mentioned it to my supervisor' as September gradually loomed, I started realise he was serious. My stress that 'I'm the only one suffering a loss' began disappearing around that time. It's because I realised he was willing to bear a fair share of burden. <7>

I decided to take childcare leave because I thought it was wrong to one-sidedly impose the burden on her. I didn't have to take childcare leave since there was also an option to add the private childcare service of babysitter to the nursery. I could also have asked my wife to take childcare leave again. We probably had those options. But, I felt it was irresponsible to one-sidedly impose the burden on her without using the right to take childcare leave when I also had it. I vaguely wondered if it was right to continue completely ignoring fulfilling my obligations as a father. My wife never asked me to take childcare leave. But she's the kind of person who tells me point-blank when she is unhappy. Because she complained everyday by saying 'Why do I have to be the one to always take care of the child?', I began thinking perhaps it's better if I did it than listening to complaints so often. Once, we've actually had such a heated fight that she stormed out of the house. I didn't know anything about childcare then. I didn't know where she kept nappies and I didn't know how to prepare baby food or milk, for example. She wasn't the type of person who is good at childcare and housework to begin with; she is the kind of person who would rather work. We are both in the same line of work and she values work as much as I do. I began thinking that it is indeed wrong for me to be working without a care in the world when she was raising our child by sacrificing her work. I also felt that I wasn't fulfilling my duty as a father to my child. I must have really felt that I owed something after being told many things by my wife. So I took childcare leave.

Because I'm on childcare leave, I'm doing all housework and childcare now. I've accepted that this is the way it is. I mean, it was the other way around before. When she was on childcare leave, I rarely did anything. I don't wish her to do housework or childcare. I mean, I'm on childcare leave to do housework and childcare. I think my wife naturally expects that. I'm sure she's probably thinking 'That's what I did before. It's your turn'. <8>

3. On the stage in which the husband returns to work:

In the long run, I think the burden of childcare will probably be fifty-fifty. So, I think it's okay if the burden on me will be larger than on my husband for about a year after he returns to work. <7>

I can't think about after returning to work. How will things be after April? I'm completely preoccupied about whether my kid will get used to the nursery, what I should do when he becomes sick, and how two of us will manage picking him up at the nursery at a specific time. Then again, to raise a child while both of us work at the kind of jobs that we have, we just have to try to make it work out even if it seems almost impossible. I could transfer to a department that is not as busy. In fact, I'm thinking that I'd better consider it as well. But I don't know if I can switch departments in the way I want. There are so many unknowns after April. <8>

4. On the post-transfer stage, occurring after about four months since the husband's reinstatement:

I used to think 'I'm the only one at loss. It's not fair. It's not right'. But my husband took childcare leave and, after returning to work, voluntarily requested and transferred to a department where time is relatively more flexible. Since he gave up something as well, I feel thankful and also somewhat guilty. So, the stress 'I'm the only one losing out' has been reduced considerably. It's not that I'm the only one suffering a loss. My husband used to work hard until midnight immediately after returning to work. Even though he was all energetic outside, by the time he came home, he would be so exhausted that he couldn't even talk. That wasn't good for him and I was also very unhappy thinking 'I'm losing out when he's doing what he likes'. The stress that I felt then was enormous. Now, he comes home early, too. Since we can sit down and talk at night, I'm much less stressed in that sense.

I think my husband is happy now. But I'm sure he has a dilemma, too. He wanted to climb up the corporate ladder and has done just that. He has been doing his job steadily. I think he probably dwells on the fact he is away from the frontline, albeit temporarily. That said, before he transferred, he was in the state in which he couldn't even talk when I asked him how his day was because he was completely exhausted. Now, he says things like 'I want to do something like this' or 'oh, this is interesting'. He probably comes up with ideas because his brain isn't as tired. I think you can work longer when you work in a way to still have enough energy to think about ideas for work when you come home than working in a way that you can't even talk when you are done working. I think you are happier that way, too.

I think one should be responsible for one's own career. If my husband wants to go back to his old department two years from now, I think he should go ahead. If he decides to go back, well, I'll do what I can do. I'll ask him to find a way to bear a fair share of burden to the best of his ability. If he goes back to his old department, we won't be able to share housework and childcare in the way we do now. I think we just have to come up with a new way to work while sharing housework and childcare between the two of us. But, deep down in my heart, I'm optimistic that he will transfer again to a department where it is easier to balance work and family, even if he decides to go back to his old department once. <7>

My schedule is not as tight in my current department. It's so much easier in terms of time. I can write articles and read documents in the middle of night. Since my current job allows me to manage my own time, this is better for raising a child. I could have worked more if we didn't have a child. To be honest, I do feel unhappy about it. But I adore my child. The sense of fulfilment that I get when I spend time with him is greater than the unhappiness for not being able to work because we have a child. I'm enjoying myself now that I have time to be with my child. <8>

5.4.8 Towards a Decent Work-Family Interface

5.4.8.1 Changes in Attitudes Towards Work After Taking Childcare Leave

Many individuals experienced a change in their attitude towards work after they took childcare leave. They began to question their long work hours.

When you return to work after experiencing childcare leave, you feel ridiculous working until late at night. You work until late at night because you are preparing for the worst. But is it true that we can't work unless we are prepared for the worst? No, I don't think that's necessarily true. So, I try to go home early whenever I can. <7>

I also think it is family, not work, that will be here at the end. I really enjoy working. But on the other hand, I feel 'What is the point to be up to my eyes in work like this?' Every day, when I come home and see my children's faces, I'm just filled with love and think 'What is the use of spending so much time on work?' <9>

Subject <8>, a male who took childcare leave, stated that he began to feel the desire to seek a better balance between work life and family life after he took childcare leave. His wife noticed that change in his attitude as well. She was highly satisfied with the change in her husband's attitude.

I'm not satisfied with the way my husband does housework. However, I'm very happy with how he cares for the child. For example, when our son suddenly wakes up and cries out at night, my husband springs to his feet to cradle the child. So, I do feel I have to overlook his housework to some extent. I do more housework than him. He does more childcare than me. I think he's very engaged in childcare largely because he has taken childcare leave. He has changed a lot after taking childcare leave. I think he reluctantly took childcare leave at the beginning. But he probably began feeling affection as he took care of the child. Even after he returned to work, he tries to come home while our son is still awake, for example. He used to go for a drink with his colleagues after work, even after our son was born. He wasn't trying to participate in childcare. It seems experiencing childcare leave prompted him to become more proactive about raising the child. <7>

5.4.8.2 Establishing a New Way of Working

There are some companies that strive to create a scheme in which their professional employees can work shorter hours. This was also beneficial from the perspective of increasing the choices available to workers. Subjects <7> and <15>, who were both regarded as model cases, understood this benefit and planned to balance their own career goals with their companies' aims, because it not only help the themselves, but also those who are thinking of choosing the 'dual-earner couples with children' approach.

I'm trying not to work too hard because if I do, people who follow suit will be expected to work hard as well. Naturally, I'm conscious that I'm the one to establish vested interests that one can only do so much when she/he is working while raising a child. On the other hand, I'm sure there are people who want to work hard even after having a child. So, for the sake of those people, I absolutely cannot get a black mark saying 'those with children are useless (i.e., they cannot handle important tasks) as expected'. Personally, I do wonder whether I should prioritise work or family. I'm trying to balance 'not working too hard' and 'performing decent job'. <7>

I'm the oldest of all the women in my department. There are many female co-workers who are younger than me and it's highly likely that they will face the same situation in the future. They will end up working while raising children. If I fail now, they'll probably think 'Oh no, this company isn't good. I can't keep working at this company'. I'm sure my boss is worried about that as well; worried about whether I will succeed now and worried that the company will disappoint my junior co-workers if I fail. My boss seems to think

> it will be a problem if my case doesn't go well. I'm the first one who works by actually utilising the childcare-break system. My boss helps me by communicating to the management department the issues that surface as the system is put into practice. If he thinks the issue that I pointed out is indeed problematic, he talks to the management department by saying 'we should improve these aspects'. It helps me. In short, the problem is that I cannot be paid for overtime. After discussing it with my boss and getting a buy-in from him, I've been working while balancing out the total work hours by going home early to make up for the overtime work. My boss and I thought about what to do with a system for tracking the total work hours. And we decided to submit a monthly report on the frequency and status of incidents when my work hours did not coincide with the regular work hours of 9:30 a.m. to 4:30 p.m. We decided to submit a report on actual numbers of pluses (overtime) and minuses (shortened work hours) when all work hours are summed up for a given month. We arranged it so that the management department can understand the difficult situations that arise when you actually work under the childcare-break system. <15>

5.4.8.3 The Need for a 'Decent Track'

Companies 'would prefer that all employees were willing to give their all to the company' (Schwartz 1989). However, some subjects remarked that the problem lies with the fact that a method of work that prioritises family has not been established as a choice for regular employees. The need for a career track that could be called a 'decent track' was observed among men as well. Otherwise, it might happen that individuals come to decide to not have (additional) children because they have already reached their limit of work.

> If we had tried to have a child by taking the work schedule into consideration, we might not have gotten pregnant. It's very possible for us to have kept saying things like 'next year then' and 'once this project is done' and ended up not having a child. Seriously, if you think about balancing it with work, you can't have a baby. I think it's highly likely that we end up not having another baby. First, when having one child now is already a job in itself, having another one will make childcare really hard. Next, I'm working while raising only one child, but my workplace is already accommodating me in terms of workload and it's already evoking envy around me. Given that kind of a situation, I think I'll come under more pressure at work if I have another child. Besides, after doing this job a little over ten years, the work is becoming interesting now. I'm not sure if having another child will be a plus in terms of my career development. <7>

> Ambitious people who are on the way to climb up the ladder can go ahead and marry their jobs and work at overcapacity at the expense of their private life. Meanwhile, I wish the company provided decent career paths for those who think 'I've had it with the promotion competition. I want to prioritise my family' and want to change their path. I think the promotion rate and salary for those people can be reduced. Instead, well, I wish they would create a career path to work as an expert. I don't think it's a bad idea for the company to provide a path in which employees are allowed to work as experts, such as techie, engineer, and professional clerk, even when they move away from the promotion path. My opinion is that not all corporate employees need to climb up the ladder. <12>

Here, Subject <12> mentioned a new track in which employees work as experts in their field without receiving promotion, which allows them to prioritise their family lives. This kind of track is the antonym of the fast track, in which employees must always face keen and endless competition in order to climb up the ladder.

We can call this track the 'decent track'. Those on the decent track are free from competition, work shorter hours, and receive decent salary.

The decent track shares many similarities with the 'mommy track',[5] which had its origin in Schwartz (1989) and was given its name by Lewin (1989). Although there was only a two-month time lag between Schwartz and Lewin, by the time this new track was coined the 'mommy track', it has become regarded as something very dangerous. The typical explanation was that it caused women with family responsibilities to be shunted into dead-end, low-paying jobs (Eikhof 2012).

However, in my view, Schwartz's (1989) principal aim was not to lock women out of executive positions, but to show an example of how to manage the diversity of women in the workplace in a better way, by placing 'every working woman on a continuum that runs from total dedication to career at one end to a balance between career and family at the other' (Schwartz 1989: 68).

Do all full-time employees aim to climb the corporate ladder with the condition that it requires them to devote themselves almost wholly to the companies and to compete, intensely and endlessly, with their colleagues? The fast track, or the *sogo-shoku* course in Japanese companies (Strober and Chan 2001), offers employees the possibility of promotion to the senior positions, in return for sacrificing their lives outside of the workplace. By contrast, the decent track offers opportunities for employees to have meaningful lives outside of the workplace, in return for sacrificing the possibility of promotion.

It seems that we confuse two problems. The first problem is that women, especially married mothers, are excluded from the fast track. The other problem is that employers regard only the fast track as the official course. At first, companies let ambitious women enter and go through the fast track. However, they should also offer the decent track as an official option, respecting it as an indispensable track for the company and regarding it as having the same equivalent importance as the fast track. Both tracks should be open to all employees, regardless of their gender or marital status and family status.

In Japanese companies, as we have seen in Chap. 4, while *sogo-shoku* employees are rushing about their jobs, the daily reoccurring and continuous problems in the workplace are settled by *ippan-shoku* workers. Although their contribution is still invisible to their employers, it is plausible to say that they are already indispensable in the Japanese workplace. There seems to be no reason for the employers to not to establish the decent track alongside the fast track. For them, the decent track workers will bring a decent outcome at decent cost. In turn, from the employees view, the decent track offers a decent return at decent cost; that is, the workers receive a sufficient wage to support their own lives without being forced to sacrifice their private lives.

---

[5]Many use 'mommy', whereas some did 'mummy'. For example, Eikhof (2012) uses the latter.

References

Barnett, Rosalind C. 1996. *Toward a review of the work/family literature*. Boston, MA: Wellesley College Center for Research on Women.

Bigner, Jerry J. 1994. *Individual and family development: a life-span interdisciplinary approach*. Englewood Cliffs, NJ: Prentice Hall.

De Klerk, Marissa, Alewyn Nel Jan, and Elleen Koekomoer. 2012. Positive side of the work-family interface: A theoretical review. *Journal of Psychology in Africa* 22(4): 683–694.

Demerouti, Evangelia, Maria C.W. Peeters, and Beatrice I.J.M. van der Heijden. 2012. Work-family interface from a life and career stage perspective: the role of demands and resources. *International Journal of Psychology* 47(4): 241–258.

Duvall, Evelyn Millis, and Brent C. Miller. 1985. *Marriage and family development* (6th ed). New York: Harper & Row.

Eikhof, Doris Ruth. 2012. A double-edged sword: twenty-first century workplace trends and gender equality. *Gender in Management: An International Journal* 27(1): 7–22.

Erikson, Janet Jacob, Giuseppe Martinengo, and E. Jeffrey Hill. 2010. Putting work and family experiences in context: differences by family life stage. *Human Relations* 63(7): 955–979.

Fukumaru, Yuka. 2000. Tomobataraki setai-no fufu-niokeru tajuyakuwari-to yokuutsudo-no kanren (Relationships between multiple roles of dual-career couples and depression). *Kazoku Shinrigaku Kenkyu (The Japanese Journal of Family Psychology)* 14(2): 151–162 (in Japanese).

Galinsky, Ellen. 1987. *The Six stages of parenthood*. Reading, MA: Da Capo.

Greenhaus, Jeffrey. 2008. Innovations in the study of the work-family interface: Introduction to the special section. *Journal of Occupational and Organizational Psychology* 81: 343–348.

Kanai, Atsuko. 2010. Hataraku josei-no kyaria-toranjishion (Career transition among working women). *Nihon Rodo Kenkyu Zassi (The Monthly Journal of the Japan Institute of Labour)* 603: 44–53 (in Japanese).

Kato, Yoko. 2010. *Waku Famiri Konfurikuto-no Taisho Purosesu (The coping process of Work-family Conflict)*. Kyoto: Nakanishiya Shuppan (in Japanese).

Lewin, Tamar. 1989. 'Mommy Career Track' sets off a furor. New York Times, March 8: A18.

Nicholson, Nigel. 1987. The transition cycle: a conceptual framework for the analysis of change and human resources management. *Research in Personnel and Human Resources Management: A Research Annual* 5: 209–264.

Schein, Edgar H. 1978. *Career dynamics: matching individual and organizational needs*. Reading, MA: Addison-Wesley.

Schnittger, Maureen H., and Gloria W. Bird. 1990. Coping among dual-career men and women across the family life cycle. *Family Relations* 39(2): 199–205.

Schwartz, Felice N. 1989. Management women and the new facts of life. *Harvard Business Review* 89(1): 65–76.

Senda, Yukiko. 2006. Shutoken-no tomobataraki fufu-ni okeru 'work-family interface': Ikujikyugyo shutokuchu, go-no 2-jiten-no intabyu chosa-wo motoni (The reality of work-family interface of dual career couples in the metropolitan areas: comparison of interview data taken during and after childcare leave period). In *Shoshika-no Shinkyokumen-to Kazoku, Rodo Seisaku-no Taio-ni kansuru Kenkyu* (Research on Policy Planning and Evaluation/ Health Labour Sciences Research Grant (H14-Seisaku-029), ed. Takahashi, Shigesato, 82–95 (in Japanese).

Strober, Myra H., and Agnes Milling Kaneko Chan. 2001. *The road winds uphill all the way: gender, work, and family in the United States and Japan*. Cambridge, Mass.: MIT Press.

Super, D.E. 1980. A life-span, life-space approach to career development. *Journal of Vocational Behavior* 16: 282–298.

Tanaka, Sigeto. 2003. Danjo kyodo sankaku shakai-no jitsugen kanousei: Seikatsu jikan deta-ni motozuku seisaku hyoka. *Kikan Kakei Keizai Kenkyu* 60: 48–56 (in Japanese).

Trost, Jan. 1974. This family life cycle: An impossible concept? *International Journal of Sociology of the Family*, 4, 37–47.

Voydanoff, Patricia. 2002. Linkages between the work–family interface and work, family, and individual outcomes. *Journal of Family Issues* 23: 138–164.

Williams, Kevin J., and George M. Alliger. 1994. Role stressors, mood spillover, and perceptions of work-family conflict in employed parents. *Academy of Management Journal* 37: 837–868.

Chapter 6
Concluding Remarks

More than the previous generations, the Japanese women born in the 1960s have walked a life that gave greater priority to occupational careers than to marriage and childbearing. As seen in Chap. 2, the cohort from the 1960s was the first to show a low fertility rate due to delaying pregnancy attempts. While the number of pregnancy attempts drastically dropped during their 20s, it did not increase during their 30s. It is plausible to say that they ran out of time; they put off having children throughout their 20s, along with delaying their social life-cycle, and also gave up childbirth once they were past the age deemed ideal by the social norms of the time. Although the social life-cycle began lagging behind that of previous generations, the reproduction process among women in the 1960s cohort was still defined by the deadlines imposed by social norms of the time. The 1960s cohort was one in which women's birth behaviour was extremely inactive.

The slipping in the social life-cycle made it far more acceptable for women of the 1960s cohort to work compared to prior cohorts. Therefore, in an effort to explain the change in fertility behaviour among these women, their employment behaviour was focused on. As seen in Chap. 3, the women in the 1960s cohort experienced a new balance between work and family. In the 1980s, Japan ratified the Committee on the Elimination of Discrimination against Women (CEDAW) and enacted the Equal Employment Opportunity Law (EEOL). During this period, the members of the 1960s cohort were in their twenties. It was a time of increasing momentum towards changing the conventional sexist labour environment and aiming for gender equality in the workplace. These changes gave women the genuine option to continue their occupational careers. Then, the slogan '80-year life expectancy', and the raising of the age criteria for late childbearing to 35 loosened the age norms. As a result, choices, such as marrying late or never marrying, came to be accepted as realistic options. The average age at first marriage increased, and the existence of women in their 30s who had never married ceased to be uncommon. The timing for having children was also delayed, pushing the age of a mother's first childbirth to their late 20s. In this way, changes in aforementioned

Y. Senda, *Childbearing and Careers of Japanese Women Born in the 1960s*,
Population Studies of Japan, DOI 10.1007/978-4-431-55066-2_6

social conditions gave women more freedom in choosing their life course, both in terms of their occupational career options for how long to continue working and their family career options for marriage and childbirth.

As seen in Chap. 4, when female employees were working under the course-based system, almost all of them were in the *ippan-shoku* course. Although employers expected short-term service from them, and they by themselves did not expect to serve long-term, the fact that a number of women served for many years cannot be ignored. Experiences such as being assigned more important jobs often drove career development for these women. However, only single women received such opportunities. If a woman stayed single, she had a chance of getting a rewarding job in a comfortable workplace, and earning sufficient income for living life as a single person. A recent study indicates that this is also the case for female *sogo-shoku* employees (Ouchi 2014). Ouchi showed that only those who were single, or at least married without children, had the same chance of receiving a promotion as their male colleagues. For female workers, marital and family status, especially the former, determined their occupational opportunities. Under such conditions, nothing pushed them to marry and change their lives. Kawaguchi (2005) analysed the *Japanese Panel Survey of Consumers* and found that women were strongly penalised in terms of wages when they married or became mothers. While the penalty for motherhood was still widely observed in many developed societies, the marriage penalty was unusual (Kawaguchi 2005: 53). The strong wage penalty for marriage could be due to the fact (explained in this book) that whether a woman was married or single determined the kinds of assignments she received at work, which might propel career development.

However, as shown in the M-shaped curve, most women, even those working today, married and left their jobs when they decided to have a baby. This is because it was as difficult to continue working while raising a child as ever, as seen in Chap. 5. When it came to managing the full-time jobs of both spouses and childcare, it was barely possible for a couple to manage a 24-h day, even if they each adjusted their work schedules, did less housework, and used a nursery. Striving to cope with the demands of both work and family was extremely stressful, and required enormous physical strength, which took a toll on their mental and physical health. Although they were, essentially, satisfied with this lifestyle, felt positive about it, and intended to continue it, they occasionally had moments of weakness, expressed with thoughts like 'I just can't do anymore!' or 'We may not be able to keep this lifestyle going!'

To summarize the characteristics of the 1960s cohort, we should focus on the emergence of 'work-centred'[1] women, who happened to neither marry nor have children, but instead continue to work full-time. To be sure, the majority of women in that cohort were 'family-centred' women, who married, had children, and quit their jobs (and later re-entered the labour market as non-regular workers).

[1]Hakim (2000) uses the same terminology to describe the same situation. However, the difference lies between us. She focuses on the predetermined preference and I focus on the result.

There were also a few 'work-family balancing' women, who managed to continue their full-time work alongside raising children. However, they were not characteristic of the 1960s cohort. The family-centred life course already comprised the vast majority of the 1950s and earlier cohorts. The earlier cohorts also contained women following the work-family balancing life course, since the rate of continued regular employment was constantly at about 20 % during the late-20th century (Chap. 3). In contrast, those women walking the work-centred life course were a very small minority in the earlier cohorts. For the 1960s cohort, they first became visible as a social category containing a considerable number of people that earned social acceptance as a lifestyle for women.

Note that women were not divided into the three life courses at the beginning of their life. Rather, they first began to work unanimously around the 1980s, and diversified their life courses afterwards in accordance with the conditions they faced. In this respect, their life courses were characterised as 'work-precedence' in the beginning. Because the old social norms had been changing, they needed to decide their life course on their own. Even the timing of life choices depended on their own decisions. It was a matter of course that there was a delay in the timing of life events such as marriage and childbirth. As a result, this cohort witnessed a considerable delay in their social life-cycle.

The work-family balancing life course was still unpopular for that cohort. Changes in the Japanese workplace in the mid-1980s due to the anti-discrimination law and public opinions advocating gender equality might have attracted women entering the labour force. However, in reality, there were not any sufficient measures for facilitating a work-family balance when women began to consider marriage and having a child. Simultaneous work-family balance was thus possible for only those who happened to be under favourable conditions (Abe 2005) or those who made an unbelievable effort (Nozaki 2011) (Chap. 5). Furthermore, even for those who succeeded in pursuing a simultaneous work-family balance, there were still some penalties issued in their occupational career because they did not devote themselves as companies requested. This may be a reason why the work-family balancing life course was not attractive to the majority. If one stayed single, she could go ahead. However, if she had a child, she seemed it would be better to quit the job than to struggle for work-family balance. The 'decent track', alongside of the fast track, should be provided. Otherwise, people would give up births because they were already fully busy enough.

The younger cohorts are following the same line as the 1960s cohort. Marriage rates continue to decline. Fertility is decreasing for women in their 20s. Recently, women in their 30s and 40s have shown a slight increase in their age-specific fertility (*Vital Statistics*). This means the social life-cycle continues to be delayed. Given that there are biological factors that predispose pregnancy attempts in the late 30s and 40s to infertility or miscarriage (Chap. 2), the delay in the social life-cycle will prevent a recovery from the current levels of low fertility. The experiences of the 1960s cohort, to which we referred in this book, offer valuable lessons for Japan, and for other societies under similar conditions.

References

Abe, Masahiro. 2005. Dare-ga ikujikyugyo-wo shutoku surunoka. In *Kosodate Setai-no Shakaihosho*, ed. National Institute of Population and Social Security Research, 243–264. Tokyo: University of Tokyo Press (in Japanese).

Hakim, Chatherine. 2000. *Work-lifestyle choices in the 21st century: Preference theory*. New York: Oxford University Press.

Kawaguchi, Akira. 2005. Kekkon-to shussan-wa danjo-no chingin-ni donoyona eikyo-wo oyoboshite iruka. *Nihon Rodo Kenkyu Zassi (The Monthly Journal of the Japan Institute of Labour)* 535: 42–55 (in Japanese).

Nozaki, Yuko. 2011. Waku raifu anbaransu-wa doko-de okiteiruka: Shussan penaruti-to josei-no shugyo keizoku. In *Waku raifu baransu-to kazoku keisei (Work-life balance and family formation: Changing Japanese working life)*, eds. Higuchi Yoshio, and Tetsuo Fukawa, 85–104. Tokyo: University of Tokyo Press (in Japanese).

Ouchi, Akiko. 2014. Kigyo-wa honki-de josei-wo sogo-shoku-tosite sodatete kitaka? (Have female core workers really been trained to become managers in Japan?). *Nihon Romu Gakkaishi* 15(1): 97–106 (in Japanese).

MIX
Papier aus verantwortungsvollen Quellen
Paper from responsible sources
FSC® C105338

If you have any concerns about our products,
you can contact us on
ProductSafety@springernature.com

In case Publisher is established outside the EU,
the EU authorized representative is:
Springer Nature Customer Service Center GmbH
Europaplatz 3, 69115 Heidelberg, Germany

Printed by Libri Plureos GmbH
in Hamburg, Germany